D1579924

PREVENTION BOOK

DR ROSY DANIEL
with Rachel Ellis

THE CANCER PREVENTION BOOK

The Holistic Plan to Reduce
Your Risk of Cancer and
Revolutionize Your Life

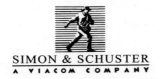

SIMON & SCHUSTER
A VIACOM COMPANY

First published in Great Britain by
Simon & Schuster UK Ltd, 2001
A Viacom Company

1 3 5 7 9 10 8 6 4 2

Simon & Schuster UK Ltd
Africa House
64–78 Kingsway
London WC2B 6AH

Simon & Schuster Australia
Sydney

A CIP catalogue record for this book is available
from the British Library

ISBN 0-7432-0940-0

Typeset by Palimpsest Book Production Limited
Polmont, Stirlingshire
Printed and bound in Great Britain by
Bath Press, Bath

The information and statistics contained in this book come from
mainstream cancer charities and orthodox medical institutions.
The views expressed are those of Dr Rosy Daniel and not
Rachel Ellis, the *Daily Express* or Simon & Schuster.
For individual advice on matters raised in this book you should
always consult either your own GP or a reliable holistic doctor.

This book is dedicated to all the people with cancer that I have worked with. They have shown me the power of the holistic approach to health through many remarkable recoveries and have convinced me of its essential role in preventing cancer for all of us.

Acknowledgements

I would like to acknowledge with deep gratitude the support of His Royal Highness the Prince of Wales for the work of the Bristol Cancer Help Centre and for his support of this work on the holistic approach to cancer prevention. The example set by the Prince both in relation to organic farming and his rejection of genetic modification are a tremendous source of encouragement to all who seek to promote personal responsibility towards the environment and healthcare.

My most sincere thanks go to Helen Gummer, my editor at Simon & Schuster, for her commissioning this book and her encouragement throughout the writing process. I would like to acknowledge the vital role played by the *Daily Express*, and particularly Sue McGeever, in supporting this project and in helping to publicize this important information on cancer prevention. Huge thanks also go to Rachel Ellis, Health Editor of the *Daily Express* until December 2000, who worked tirelessly with me to improve the original manuscript and make it more accessible to a far wider readership. Special thanks are also due to the Bristol Cancer Help Centre for its support of this project and particularly Chris Head, Pat Turton, Helen Cooke and Caroline Morrison for their invaluable feedback. I would also like to honour the very great contribution made to cancer care by the Centre's founders, Penny Brohn and Pat Pilkington since the Centre's opening in 1980 and also to honour the role of Jane Sen in revolutionizing the Centre's approach to healthy eating. Her *Healing Foods Cookbook* is a total delight and is just as applicable to the prevention of cancer as to its treatment. My warmest thanks also go to Professor Karol Sikora and Doctor Victor Barley for supporting and encouraging my role in making the holistic approach to cancer treatment and prevention more widely known and understood within conventional medical circles.

I am greatly indebted to Dr Stan Venitt, retired Emeritus Reader in Cancer Studies in the Institute of Cancer Research, University of London, for his meticulous guidance in the section 'What is Cancer' in chapter one and to Professor Sir Richard Doll, Professor of Medicine at Oxford University for his expert guidance on the causes of cancer. I was also helped enormously by the work of Professor Gabriel Kune, author of *Reducing the Odds: A Manual for the Prevention of Cancer*; Theo Colburn, Dianne Dumanoski and John Peterson Myers, authors of *Our Stolen Future*; David Steinman and Sam Epstein, authors of *The Safe Shopper's Bible*; and Suzannah Olivier, author of *The Breast Cancer Prevention and Recovery Book*, all of whom I have quoted extensively.

I would also like to express my deep gratitude to Reg Flower, Angela Burns, Lynda McGilvray, Zoe Lindgren and Mair Hoskins for sharing their personal cancer stories and their vulnerability with us in this book. This is not a step to be taken lightly and their courage in doing this is valued immensely because of the extra depth and meaning which their examples bring to the work. My most sincere thanks go to the wonderful, generous Sarah Collins and her team of volunteers for the typing of the manuscript, Katharine Young and the marvellous production team at Simon & Schuster and the excellent copyeditor Annie Bridges who pulled the work into shape so beautifully.

But most particularly, I would like to acknowledge my heartfelt gratitude for the great patience, constant encouragement and unfailing support of Danny Kustow throughout the writing of this book – and especially for his help and the help of my wonderful children, Sophie and Elouise, in retaining my sense of humour!

Rosy Daniel

CONTENTS

FOREWORD

ST. JAMES'S PALACE

The Cancer Prevention Book is a remarkable testimony to the enlightened vision of Dr. Rosy Daniel. It tells us not only many of the causes and details of how cancer develops, but also describes some of the things we can all do to help prevent cancer in our own lives. The book has been created both because of twenty years of holistic work with cancer patients at the Bristol Cancer Help Centre and the personal pain and distress Dr. Daniel has experienced as an holistic cancer doctor, watching so many lives devastated by the disease which has impelled her to take action.

Dr. Daniel's courageous work with cancer patients has shown us that cancer, one of our most feared diseases, can be turned around or slowed down, even in its advanced stages. She is now taking an even bolder step to try to take on the prevention of cancer in society as a whole. As a longtime Patron of the Bristol Cancer Help Centre, I am so glad that she has taken this initiative to bring the holistic approach to cancer out into the public arena in an attempt to enable us all to experience the health benefits associated with the Centre's approach, without having to become victims of cancer to do so.

Heartened by the results achieved at Bristol and alarmed by the fact that cancer is currently affecting four in ten people in developed countries – and rising – this book represents a really serious attempt by Rosy Daniel to persuade us all to wake up to the gravity of the situation and take personal and collective responsibility for turning the situation around.

Her point is quite simple – if cancer can be stabilised and the prognosis extended by use of the holistic approach to health for cancer patients, why not use this approach to prevent cancer in the first place? She has been so encouraged by the profound transformations in health and happiness she has witnessed over the years at Bristol, that she is now determined to apply this approach "further back down the river" to help many more of us to experience far better physical, emotional and spiritual health whilst simultaneously reducing our personal cancer risk.

Bristol has based its successful approach on the holistic health principles of working to improve the health of people with cancer at all the levels of mind, body and spirit. Since the Centre's founding in 1980 by the remarkable Penny Brohn and Pat

Pilkington, science has begun, step by step, to vindicate their entirely intuitive approach to fighting and healing cancer. The Bristol emphasis on fruit and vegetables is increasingly accepted as part of orthodox cancer prevention, and the importance of the mind-body connection in health is becoming established through the new science of psychoneuro-immunology. Even the art of visualising positive outcomes during chemotherapy has been shown to extend survival time with breast cancer. But deeper than this, by helping individuals to tackle the question of the underlying state of their spirit, their relationship to themselves and by rekindling their fundamental purpose and joy in living, enormous and often unexpected improvements in health, well-being and quality of life have been achieved.

Recently the science of epidemiologists, Sir Richard Doll and Sir Richard Peto, has shown us clearly that cancer, in part, is a lifestyle-related disease which is aggravated by environmental pollution. Our Western disregard for Nature, combined with the emotional and spiritual vacuum often caused by twentieth century living has placed us all at very great and increasing risk. It is gradually becoming clear that smoking, poor diet, stress, pollution and sedentary lifestyles are major contributing causes of cancer. Rather like the Sorcerer's Apprentice, we have in some ways been conducting a vast experiment that has begun to go seriously wrong in many aspects of our existence.

In this excellent book Dr. Daniel gives us clear guidance on how, as individuals, we may re-establish our lives based on loving, compassionate and respectful relationships to ourselves, others and our environment, returning gradually to lives with meaning and purpose. In obtaining proper support and help to re-orientate ourselves in this way to lifestyles which properly nourish and fulfil us at every level, she asserts that our bad habits will give us up as opposed to the other way round!

I have long been a wholehearted supporter of Dr. Daniel's vision of a world where cancer is a rarity and not the norm and of her dedicated effort to make a real difference in the world to improve our health and to reduce the level of human suffering.

The Cancer Prevention Book gives a vital and urgent message to all of us that cancer can be a preventable disease and tells us that it is time for us all to invest pro-actively in the protection of our health rather than becoming passive victims of serious illness. I hope this inspiring book will help to encourage us to rise to this challenge, following the example of the marvellous Bristol patients and see if we can take up and practise all the good habits suggested by Rosy Daniel.

INTRODUCTION

Cancer is now a huge problem worldwide, touching the lives of almost everyone in Western society. While the desperate search for a cure and better treatment goes on, it is clear we simply cannot wait for medical research to provide the answer. Instead, we must urgently turn our attention to the prevention of cancer through our own active and positive efforts.

Most people feel very scared of cancer but seem to think that, apart from giving up smoking, there is very little they can do to reduce their risk of getting the disease. This couldn't be further from the truth. In the pages that follow, you will learn exactly what causes cancer, and will no doubt be surprised to see that, just like heart disease, it is in the main a lifestyle-related disease. This means that if we change our lifestyle and habits, we can considerably reduce the risk of cancer. Medicine is progressing all the time, and, hopefully, there will be exciting breakthroughs in cancer treatment within our lifetimes. But meanwhile there is so much that we can be doing to improve the situation if we start taking our health and the precious gift of life seriously.

So many of us live our lives in unfulfilled, insecure, stressed states, in a vicious cycle of self-destructive attitudes and behaviours, feeling unsatisfied by the way our lives and relationships are working out. This is often the result of an emotional and spiritual vacuum in many people's lives, created through the breakdown of their community and family life or simply by having focused on the wrong priorities long term, whilst at the same time failing to nourish their personal spirit. Often, the loneliness, boredom, fear and anxiety created leads them to find solace in unhealthy food, cigarettes and alcohol. The damaging effects of these substances are greatly exaggerated by a sedentary lifestyle and extreme stress. Because it is these self-destructive behaviours which are largely to blame for cancer, it is therefore not a huge leap to see cancer indirectly as an emotional or spiritual problem which needs to be addressed at all levels of our being.

Once we find ourselves in low-energy, demotivated states, there is a real inertia or 'stuckness'. We may know what is good or bad for us but be quite unable to do anything about it. What is needed then is a great deal of support and encouragement; and, most important of all, we need to start to feel good about ourselves and our lives again. Finding a way out of the inertia trap is the essence of the holistic approach to health, which is based on the idea that our health degenerates as a result of spiritual malaise and that the ability to make healthy changes is linked to the state of our body, mind and spirit. Getting the right levels of emotional support, guidance, encouragement and uplift to our spirit is really the only way to make good sustainable changes in our behaviour possible.

Until now, most health promotion campaigns have been based around the dissemination of information, but information alone cannot change the state of an individual who is 'stuck'. By contrast, the holistic approach to health recognizes that it is vital to work first with our emotional state, to rekindle our energy, enthusiasm, and most fundamentally, our will to live and sense of purpose. Following on rapidly from this is the crucial need to develop self-esteem and a new protective, nurturing relationship towards ourselves. Only then is it possible to start changing the way we lead our lives.

But first, some understanding of what cancer is, what causes it and who is at risk is needed. It is also necessary to understand the current situation with regard to conventional cancer medicine and research and the politics surrounding them in order to appreciate the real urgency of the situation. Whilst this all makes somewhat depressing reading, the aim is to put you fully in the picture so that you can see how vital it is for you to get involved personally in the prevention of cancer – both for yourself and society as a whole.

The first three chapters of this book take an in-depth look at cancer, how common it is, its causes, its risk factors and how to reduce them, and how relatively ineffective medicine is at treating the disease. Chapters 4, 5 and 6 will show you the other, more positive, side of the story.

Every form of cancer has been shown, on occasions, to regress or even disappear completely from the body, even after medical treatment has been deemed ineffective. This can happen by spontaneous remission (when the cancer simply disappears from the body), which can be made more likely by adopting the holistic approach to health in the presence of illness. The process of remission shows that the body does have a mechanism for dealing with cancer and that cancer need not be the death sentence so many people perceive it to be.

In healthy people, many hundreds of cancer cells are made every day which are either repaired or destroyed through the cells' DNA protective mechanisms or the body's immune surveillance. It is when these in-built mechanisms for recognizing and dealing with cancer break down that cancer can develop and grow in the body.

Even in people who have cancer, the body's protective systems work at very different levels of effectiveness. We know this because there are enormous variations in the time it takes for cancer to spread and for a secondary cancer to appear in different people with the same type of cancer. Sometimes, secondary cancers develop within six months or a year of first being diagnosed, while in other cases this can take as long as twenty years.

Whilst in part this time difference is due to the grade or aggressiveness of the tumour, it is also due to the level of host resistance, or quite simply the body's ability to fight back. In cases of cancer remission it is clear that the body's defence system has become active and effective again. Preventing cancer basically involves understanding and building up these defence mechanisms rather than blindly subjecting ourselves to things which destroy the body's ability to cope and stay well.

The book is divided into six chapters. In Chapter 1 you will find a full explanation of cancer and its causes. If you are not so interested in the disease itself but want to find out how to tackle eliminating the main sources of cancer from your life, start reading the book at Chapter 2. Chapter 3 will alert you to the most common signs of cancer. Treating cancer early is almost another form of prevention. This is because many cancers, if treated early enough before they have spread into other parts of the body, may never cause problems again. It is wise to make yourself aware of these common symptoms so that, without getting over-anxious, you can keep an eye on yourself and your family members and know when to insist that you get a referral for proper tests or a consultant opinion.

If you want to go straight to the holistic plan to prevent cancer by achieving positive health, start reading from Chapter 4 onwards, using the factual parts of the book in Chapters 1, 2 and 3 as a reference to dip into as needed.

Overall, the main purpose of this book is to put you firmly in the driving seat of your life, in a position to achieve excellent health and a greatly enhanced sense of well-being, vitality and aliveness at all levels of mind, body and spirit. The key elements of the plan described in this book have been used by thousands of people with cancer who have attended the Bristol Cancer Help Centre, many of whom have achieved remarkable recoveries. Examples of their stories have been included to illustrate the power of the holistic approach to health in fighting cancer, which will help you to see clearly the great relevance of this approach to its prevention. But this book is not written for people with cancer – it is for those who are cancer free, who want to make sure they stay that way. My book describing the Bristol approach to cancer, called *Living with Cancer*, is more suitable for anyone who already has the disease, see Appendix 1.

Once you have read *The Cancer Prevention Book*, it is then a question of deciding which are the most important steps to take to make the biggest difference to your own personal cancer risk. As you read through the following pages, try to avoid getting overwhelmed by the sheer number of possible risk factors involved in getting cancer, a few of which you may be able to do nothing about. However, for most of us, there are usually one or two really important things we could change which could dramatically decrease our risk. Try to keep an eye out for what they might be for you, and then go about setting yourself achievable goals as described in Chapter 6, 'Getting Started'.

It is a good idea to see cancer prevention as a long-term project, introducing healthy changes bit by bit. Don't try to change everything at once because you can become overwhelmed and give up. In Chapters 2, 4 and 5, there is a lot of practical advice about how to make sustainable changes. If you stick to this advice, realizing that nearly all of our 'bad habits' represent an emotional need which must be met in another way before we are likely to be able to change, you should be able to succeed without too much difficulty. It is likely that after making these changes you will soon feel far better than you have done in a very long time. In fact, by taking the necessary steps to prevent cancer you are very likely to experience many other health benefits too.

The advice given in this book is based upon the holistic approach to cancer that has been pioneered at the

Bristol Cancer Help Centre. It is obvious both to the people who have used to the Centre's approach to fight and heal cancer and the staff who work there, that what has been learnt about tackling cancer must now be applied to help prevent it.

CHAPTER 1: GETTING THE PICTURE

THE CANCER PROBLEM

The cancer problem has now reached epidemic proportions in developed countries – four people in ten will get cancer in their lifetime and one in four will die from it. As the Western lifestyle spreads to less developed areas of the world, overtaking traditional cultures, cancer incidence in these countries is rising to match that of the West. Yet despite fifty years of intensive cancer research and vast sums of money spent, we are achieving a cure in only three of the rarer types of cancer. Only in testicular cancer, some of the leukaemias and some of the lymphomas, is cure a realistic possibility. In the four most common cancers – of the breast, lung, colon and prostate – conventional medicine can but hope to increase the 'disease free interval' rather than prolong life significantly.

What cancer research has shown us, however, is how this disease develops in the body, what causes cancer and how the incidence varies around the world depending on local cultures and differences in lifestyle. Most helpful in understanding the priorities for cancer prevention is the picture given to us by British epidemiologists Sir Richard Doll and Sir Richard Peto. Their research shows that in the West, 81.5 per cent of cancer deaths relate to lifestyle factors – 35 per cent of cancer is caused by diet, 30 per cent by smoking, 10 per cent by reproductive hormones, 5 per cent by alcohol and 1.5 per cent by physical inactivity. This leaves only 18.5 per cent of cancer deaths attributable to external or environmental factors, such as infection which causes 10 per cent, electromagnetic radiation (EMR) 4 per cent, pollution (including food additives) 2 per cent, occupational exposure to cancer-causing chemicals like asbestos 2 per cent, and medicines and medical procedures 0.5 per cent.

This is not the picture most of the public have about cancer. Generally, people are aware of the connection between smoking and cancer, but most would say the second biggest cause of cancer is environmental pollution. A connection between food and cancer is usually linked to food additives but, as the figures show, these are, along with all other forms of pollution, responsible for just 4 per cent of cancer deaths.

The commonly held belief that cancer is caused mainly by environmental pollution leaves people feeling impotent and thinking that there is precious little they can do personally to reduce the risk of cancer. But this belief is wrong. As we can see clearly from the medical evidence, cancer is a lifestyle disease. It is therefore absolutely vital that individually, socially and globally, we tackle this problem head-on and make all efforts possible to eradicate it. With a combination of key information about the causes of cancer and, most crucially, the necessary personal support and motivation to change our lifestyles, the cancer picture could be changed dramatically.

For the past fifteen years I have worked as a holistic doctor and, latterly, as Medical Director of the Bristol Cancer Help Centre. At the Centre the holistic approach to health is used to help people with cancer fight to regain their health. It has become crystal clear at Bristol that many of the steps individuals can take to promote their health, even in the presence of illness, can make a crucial difference in their efforts to stabilize the disease. Over twenty years many people who have undertaken the Centre's holistic approach have undergone such a profound revival of their health, happiness and fulfilment in life, that frequently the cry goes up as people leave Bristol of 'Why, oh why did I have to wait until I got cancer to get healthy and come alive and really experience true health in this way?'

Reg Flower was diagnosed with malignant melanoma in 1982 and found his way to the Bristol Cancer Help Centre through reading a chance article in the paper. He was immensely relieved to be given practical steps to fight his cancer through diet and complementary medicines. But it was not until a year later, when he developed secondaries a few months after being abruptly and traumatically made redundant from his work, that the deeper value of the Centre's approach really came home to him. Reg was absolutely devastated by his redundancy as he had personally twice pulled his firm back from the brink of bankruptcy and had been promised a position on the firm's board in the fullness of time. He had always been a worka-holic, putting everything he had and more into his work, covering up other people's errors or failures. He could not see how his dedication to the firm could possibly have resulted in redundancy. He was also very frightened by the recurrence of the disease and realized that something major had to change if he was going to survive.

When he returned to the Centre the first crucial thing he managed to do was to let go and express his emotions through counselling sessions. With enough support he overcame a lifetime's inhibition, weeping and raging until his hurt and anger were fully expressed. He then, to his own amazement, having always been a 'tough sort of bloke', discovered the profound benefits of spiritual healing, relax-ation and meditation. Within a short while, his perspec-tive on life changed completely. He began to regain his sense of humour, beginning to laugh at himself for having got things so dreadfully out of proportion for so many years. He just could not believe that he had allowed his work to take him over so completely. He realized what was really important to him in life and began to put time and energy into being with his wife and children. He started growing organic vegetables in his garden, and spent hours in his garage, making rocking horses for the kids rather than new prototypes for his engineering work, as he had before. But even more important, he learnt how to take time just to be with himself or simply to stop and appre-ciate the beauty of life around him. He says that after the change in his life, he would stop the car and sit for an hour or two just watching the sun go down – deeply moved by the beauty of nature and his sense of connection to it.

In the years that followed Reg started his own business and did extremely well, but he was always mindful of the necessity to keep his priorities right. At this point in 2001, he is still living, nearly twenty years after having had secondary melanoma and being told he had maybe two years more life, if he was lucky.

Reg is sure that his survival is due to his wholesale adoption of the holistic approach to health and his changed lifestyle. But his great frustration is that people have to get seriously ill to get their lives sorted out in this way. He says: 'If only people could do all this before they got ill. All I see around me is miserable-looking people rushing around in ever-decreasing circles, stressed out of their minds about some total irrelevancy, making themselves sicker and sicker in the process. Every time I get on the tube in London, I see tense unhappy faces – no one is smiling. If only they could all stop and get back to what really makes them happy and brings them alive. I had to do that, and not only has it saved my life but the pleasure I now get out of the simplest things is mind-blowing. We have to get this message across to people who are still cancer free – for God's sake stop the risky things you are doing and act now to get your priorities right. Learn from those of us who have trodden this path before you. We've been through it and learnt the hard way – you don't have to do that if you follow the holistic plan now and get your life and health back into shape!'

It has been immensely gratifying to walk this path with many thousands of people with cancer, helping them to find their mental, physical and spiritual healing. But the pain, fear and anguish caused to these individuals by this extremely nasty disease has impelled me to try to help people everywhere to employ this holistic approach to health before cancer develops. I have witnessed so many remarkable recoveries from cancer through the use of the holistic approach that it seems obvious to use it to prevent the disease arising in the first place.

People who come to the Bristol Centre describe the cancer as the most shocking 'wake up call', compelling them to completely rethink their relationship to themselves, their health and to life itself. Surely, it must be possible for all of us to wake up now and take stock of the state of our lives, health and well-being before we have to be terrified into doing so?

The aim of this book is to help those wishing to make radical improvements to their health to identify the factors that are currently compromising them and putting them at risk. It will also provide step-by-step guidance on how to get the right level of support to address and remove these obstacles so that an entirely new state of enhanced physical health and well-being can be reached. Many of us equate getting healthy with assuming a monastic lifestyle in a state of terrible deprivation! This is a great fallacy. In reality, the effects of a heavy Western diet, toxic smoke and alcohol, obesity, inactivity and boredom cause our minds and energy levels to become extremely sluggish and lead to increasingly deep apathy and unhappiness. On the other hand, the sense of aliveness and exhilaration that is experienced as we shed these layers of sedation and toxicity, live out our passion and purpose and achieve our potential in life, is quite wonderful and could not be more exciting!

In reading this book you will have the opportunity to:

- learn about cancer, its causes and the current state of cancer medicine and research.

- learn about the holistic approach to health and how to clean up your act, eliminating the potential sources of cancer in your life.

- learn how to maximize your physical health so that you become positively healthy and not just disease free.

- work to optimize the effect that your mind, spirit and lifestyle are having on your physical health.

Emphasis will be placed throughout the book on getting the emotional support to make these changes rather than merely the information about what to change: this is crucial to making any sustainable health-promoting change in your life. Before embarking on this practical step-by-step approach, it is important to first take an in-depth look at what cancer is and what causes it, since this will put all the other recommendations into perspective. But, as said earlier, if you find the technical aspects of cancer heavy-going, you could go straight to Chapter 2 which deals with the practicalities of how to reduce the cancer risk in your life.

WHAT IS CANCER?

Cancer is a disease which results from the uncontrollable growth of cells in the body – most commonly due to damage of the cells' genetic material (DNA), or other abnormalities which stimulate repeated cell division. A cancer arises from one single cell which has become abnormal and which multiplies and multiplies until a solid mass of tissue or tumour is formed. In the case of blood cancers, the blood becomes full of abnormal blood cells. Because within the body there are 200 different kinds of cells which are the starting point for all our different tissues, there are as many different types of cancer. This makes the study of cancer the most enormously complex business. However, the underlying principles of what causes healthy cells to go 'wild' and become cancerous are becoming increasingly well understood.

All cells contain a nucleus, which has in it twenty-three pairs of chromosomes. Each time a new cell is formed, these twenty-three pairs split apart and are copied, or replicated, so that a new pair of twenty-three chromosomes goes off into each daughter cell. All along these chromosomes are genes, which are sequences of informational blueprint or codes for the manufacture of every sort of tissue and chemical within the body. Cells are dividing and replicating all the time and it is estimated that in a healthy body, most of the tissues are turned over in around two months. The more dense, bony tissues have a slower turn around but are still in a constant state of flux.

DNA damage

This means that in healthy cells there is an orderly process of replication or copying of the genetic information. In order to do this, the DNA must be replicated exactly so that the two resulting cells are identical and healthy. The problem comes when errors occur in this replication process. It is estimated that faulty DNA replication only occurs in one in a million million replications, which is a miraculously low rate! When these errors do occur, one of three things can happen. Either the cell corrects the damage or it becomes so abnormal that it becomes programmed for cell death, which is called apoptosis. The third, much more dangerous thing that can happen is that the changed DNA escapes the cell's repair or suicide mechanisms and is passed to the new daughter cells and all subsequent generations of cells as division continues. These changes in the DNA which are propagated throughout subsequent cell divisions are called mutations.

This very tiny 'natural' mutation rate of cells within the human body is increased dramatically by exposure of the cells to mutagens – substances which induce genetic changes that may lead to cancer. The process is also increased by other tumour-inducing agents or physical mutagens such as cancer-causing viruses, radioactivity, and ultraviolet radiation from sunlight, as well as by the cells' own toxic waste (the by-products of cellular metabolism). The initial mutation is only the first of five or six mutational steps towards the creation of a malignant cell. It is now understood that, over time, sequential mutations accumulate in the damaged cell to the point where the cell's growth and repeated division becomes out of control. At this point the tumour formed has the potential not only to grow rapidly in the tissue of origin, but also for daughter cells to break off from the main tumour and travel in the bloodstream. These stray cells can then take up residence in other distant parts of the body, growing there as secondary cancerous tumours, known as metastases.

The process by which cancer develops, called carcinogenesis, is seen in three stages: initiation, promotion and progression. Initiation is sparked by 'initiators' or triggers (usually mutagens), which cause changes in DNA structure. Agents which cause promotion are effectively those that pour 'fuel on the fire', accelerating the growth of cancer cells. Progression is the term used for the process of a benign tumour becoming malignant. In this situation, rapid cell growth of fairly normal cells occurs but then, over time, these cells begin to turn nasty, eventually becoming a full-blown cancer. Many carcinogens, such as asbestos, can cause all three processes to occur, and are called complete carcinogens.

Some carcinogens consistently cause cancer in specific organs. A good example of this is aflatoxin B – produced by certain moulds that contaminate staple foods such as grains – which causes liver cancer. Another is asbestos, which causes cancer of the lining of the lung, called mesothelioma. It is clear that exposure to several carcinogens simultaneously can have a compound effect which is greater than the effect of individual carcinogens. For example, lung cancer is far more likely in a person who smokes and has also been exposed to asbestos.

Mutation

There are three main types of mutation which can occur spontaneously or can be caused by carcinogens. The first type is a *point mutation* where one particular bit of the genetic information is changed or deleted. Normally the code is set in groups of three 'letters' or 'bases'. So if we imagine that the gene information normally reads: 'Bob got one egg for Jim', the substitution of one letter could leave us with: 'Bob got one ego for Jim'. Clearly, the sense is lost altogether and this type of base-pair substitution accounts for many of the P53 cancer-gene effects that have been well publicized by the media (see page 22 on Tumour Suppressor Genes).

Another type of problem is caused when there is an omission of one letter (or base). By losing the letter 'o' in Bob the other letters are moved forward and we get: 'Bbg oto nee ggf orJ im'. This is called a frame shift mutation and it creates a very distorted genetic message right along the chromosome, just through the simple loss of one bit of information.

The next type of mutation is called *chromosome mutation*. This happens when chromosomes break and are reassembled in the wrong order. This type of mutation is thought to be of critical significance in cancer.

The third type is *genomic mutation*, where there is a change in the actual number of chromosomes in the nucleus. Loss or gain of a single chromosome is known as aneuploidy and this too is regarded as a very important element in the process of carcinogenesis.

DNA has many potentially reactive sites along its

structure to which other harmful chemicals can join. Among these are the dangerous reactive chemicals called 'free radicals', which can be produced within the cell itself as toxic by-products of cellular metabolism. Others include carcinogenic chemicals from the environment (such as polycyclic aromatic hydrocarbons from exhaust fumes and smoke) and many other environmental pollutants which can find their way into the cell nucleus and bind to DNA.

Once bound to DNA these chemicals are called adducts, and they play a major role in carcinogenesis. Sometimes the adducts form cross-links between the two strands of DNA, inhibiting proper replication. Adducts can be so bulky that they distort the DNA structure and cause errors during DNA replication. In other cases, due to the presence of adducts (or of different triggers, like X-rays), single and double strands of DNA break and in turn can create more free radicals. Free radicals are atoms or molecules which contain an unpaired electron that seeks out other electrons from neighbouring chemicals to attain a more stable and less reactive state. The free-radical damage caused by this process is involved in several important mechanisms of carcinogenesis, including those caused by chromium, nickel compounds and asbestos.

We now have a picture of a cell whose DNA has become mutated by an initiator and which then goes through five or six successive mutations, escaping the normal repair or suicide mechanisms of the cell, producing a new cell line that, paradoxically, has a survival advantage over the cells around it. Very often it is the genes involved in cell repair which mutate, seriously damaging the cell's ability to protect itself. Once this crucial function is lost, the cell can start to multiply out of control. The most important mutations are in genes which:

- control communication between cells – known as signal transduction.

- control the cell's growth cycles.

- maintain gene stability.

- mediate cell death – called apoptosis.

- are normally responsible for controlling the lifespan of cells.

Normally, the DNA code is checked and corrected by 'proof reading' systems during and after DNA replication. Once abnormalities are detected, division can be halted and DNA repaired. This can happen in a series of steps called:

- damage targeting

- incision

- damage removal

- resynthesis

It is when these surveillance and repair operations themselves become faulty that the trouble begins.

Genes which control cell growth cycles and genomic stability have been identified and found to be mutated in human cancer. These are often referred to as 'cancer genes', which is a useful shorthand. But it must be remembered that a cancer gene is a mutant version of a normal gene which now creates abnormal proteins itself or has become lost altogether.

GENETIC PREDISPOSITION TO CANCER

Great emphasis has been placed in the press over the past decade on the new understanding of the inherited risk of cancer and the presence of these cancer genes, or onco-genes as they are known. What must be stressed straight-away is that it is currently estimated that only between 1 and 5 per cent of all cancers come through this heredi-tary route.

Oncogenes are mutant forms of a large family of genes called proto-oncogenes. Proto-oncogenes are genes which normally control cell growth and proliferation, helping to see cells safely through their normal growth cycle. When they themselves become mutated, they become danger-ous because they fail to work effectively at monitoring cell growth.

Tumour suppressor genes

The other side of the picture is that in healthy cells there are also tumour suppressor genes, which are involved in maintaining the stability of the cells. When these become mutated themselves, again, cells are able to grow out of control. The best known of these suppressor genes is the

P53 gene. It is estimated that probably half of all cancers contain P53 mutations. The P53 gene is easily affected by carcinogens such as aflatoxin B, carcinogenic substances in tobacco smoke, vinyl chloride and chromates (used in industrial processes), and asbestos, as well as by radio-activity and ultraviolet radiation from sunlight.

Germline mutation

So far the mutations mentioned are those which happen within one person from cell to cell as cells in the body divide. This is known as 'somatic mutation'. There is also another possibility, called 'germline mutation', when mutations occur in the reproductive tissues – namely, the eggs in the ovaries or sperm in the testicles. This gives the possibility that mutations, and therefore a risk of cancer, can be passed on to the next generation. The most common inherited defects are tumour suppressor gene abnormalities. However, these are rare and by far the majority of cancers occur as a result of somatic mutations.

Overall, the risk of cancer can be classified by divid-ing the population into four groups:

- the background 'spontaneous' group, where random mutations occur in normal people.

- the environmental group, where mutations may be caused by chemicals, radiation or viruses, or a combi-nation of these factors.

- the environmental/genetic group, made up of people

who are at greater risk from exposure to carcinogens owing to what are called pharmacogenetic polymorphisms. This means they break down certain chemicals in a more dangerous way, creating by-products that are toxic to the body.

- the purely genetic group, in whom genetic susceptibility is more important than either spontaneous or environmentally induced events.

Screening for DNA damage

Genetic science has moved so fast that the entire human genome that determines human life is now completely mapped out. This means it is rapidly becoming possible for gene structure to be checked using DNA microchip technology. The whole human genome can be contained on just ten microchips! It will also soon be feasible to assess individuals for mutations in oncogenes and tumour suppressor genes, as well as checking for the presence of pharmacogenetic polymorphisms. Checks like this would alert people to their individual susceptibility to the environmental and occupational toxins that can trigger cancer, thus helping to identify those who are at increased risk. Within our lifetime, this kind of test may become a realistic part of cancer prevention.

In the workplace, monitoring of body fluids or tissues for genotoxicity and DNA adduct formation (called biomonitoring) is also becoming possible. The aim of biomonitoring is to prevent occupational cancers by giving early warning of exposure. Where occupational exposure does exist, it can be severely compounded by other factors such as smoking, diet, drugs, medical procedures and other diseases. As with environmental carcinogens, the effect of occupational chemical exposure may be exacerbated if an individual is less able to reduce the carcinogenic threat in the body. Meanwhile, industrial and medicinal chemicals are now routinely tested for their ability to damage DNA so that dangerous exposure to carcinogenic chemicals is reduced at source.

It must be stressed that there are also carcinogens which do not damage DNA. These can be:

- enzyme inducers, which speed up enzyme activity in the cell

- hormones (either made by the body or taken as medicines or from environmental pollution directly or in the form of chemicals known as endocrine disruptors)

- hormone modifying substances

- various chemically inert materials

The common factor in these types of chemicals is their ability to stimulate sustained cell division rather than damaging the DNA itself. The problem here is that rapidly dividing cells are more prone to mutation, increasing the risk that cancer may develop.

As people get older, there is also an increase in the frequency of mutation. This may account in part for the greatly increased cancer incidence in older people in comparison with children or young adults. The other important factors are:

- the build-up of free-radical damage in the DNA

- progressive failure of DNA repair

- the time needed for a particular cell lineage to accumulate the number of different mutations necessary for cancer to develop

THE GROWTH OF A CANCER

Once a cancer cell lineage has become established, its cells begin to multiply unchecked. Once the tumour growth passes a volume of 1 cubic millimetre, it requires a blood supply and starts to evolve its own capillary network. Eventually the tumour grows big enough to invade surrounding lymph and blood vessels. It is when tumour cells then break off and migrate through the lymph and blood system, that the really serious side of cancer begins.

In the early stages of tumour growth, it is sometimes possible for the immune system to eradicate tumour cells. However, tumour cells can also develop mechanisms to avoid detection by the immune system, allowing tumours to grow unchecked. When cells reach nearby lymph nodes, the body will often attempt to fight back and the lymph nodes will swell. But, in many cases, the rapidly dividing cancer cells take over the lymph nodes and the cancer spreads still further.

Simultaneously, by this stage cancer cells will have also

entered the bloodstream. These breakaway cells can become lodged in distant capillary beds in key organs within the body such as the liver, lung or brain. These cells can then begin to multiply, forming new tumours. It is at this point that the cancer can become life threatening because these secondary deposits or metastases can grow large enough to cause failure of the vital organs, severe weight loss and, in many cases, death.

WHAT CAUSES CANCER?

Within the limits of our current understanding, the main causes of cancer in developed countries, in order of seriousness and with percentage of deaths attributable, are:

- diet (35 per cent)

- smoking (30 per cent)

- reproductive hormones (10 per cent)

- infection (10 per cent)

- alcohol (5 per cent)

- electromagnetic radiation (4 per cent)

- pollution and food additives (2 per cent)

- occupational hazards (2 per cent)

- physical inactivity (1.5 per cent)

- medical procedures (0.5 per cent)

These are the percentages calculated by the British epidemiologists, Sir Richard Peto and Sir Richard Doll of Oxford University in their joint Imperial Cancer Research Fund and Medical Research Council study. The picture created by the findings of these world-renowned scientists is that cancer is a lifestyle-related disease, with environmental factors contributing only a tiny proportion to overall cancer mortality.

This view is being heavily challenged by environmentalists, who feel that the role in carcinogenesis of intensive agriculture, with its heavy reliance on the use of chemical pesticides and fertilizers, as well as that of traffic and industrial pollution, is much higher. Environmentalists also believe that the effects of intensive farming significantly reduce food quality, which in turn influences an individual's susceptibility to cancer because of the lack of key minerals in foods. There is also serious concern about the carcinogens in many common household products we all use daily.

It is vitally important that we look not only at what is proven beyond any shadow of doubt scientifically but also at newer theories which may be receiving less scientific attention. In some cases, this may be because of the great threat such research could pose to the livelihood of the farming, manufacturing, petrochemical, drug and industrial communities.

In describing the process of carcinogenesis, what becomes clear is that it is a complex multi-step process. We have heard that there are some agents (such as asbestos) which are so damaging to cell nuclei and genetic material that their influence alone can cause cancer.

However, it would appear that in the majority of cancers there is a synergistic effect of several types of factors. It is very likely that the toxic load which accumulates in the body over a lifetime from ingested pollutants, through diet or by being inhaled through the lungs, sets the stage for the chemistry of cells to become abnormal. Scientist Professor Sam Epstein, in *The Safe Shopper's Bible* (see Appendix 1), tells us that over 400 chemical contaminants have been found in the tissues of humans, and other scientists have estimated that 'healthy' British women have some 200 chemical pollutants in their breast milk!

Because of this heavy chemical load on the body, we need to know what is going on with the body's ability to eliminate these toxins, and in particular why this ability seems to have become so compromised. One of the main factors implicated is sedentary lifestyle and obesity. It is very interesting to note that physical inactivity is now included among the measurable causes of cancer. The body's cleansing mechanisms rely almost entirely on muscular activity to remove toxic waste from the tissues, and it is entirely understandable that allowing the body to become sluggish and the tissues 'stagnant' should result in higher cancer rates. What must also be considered is the fact that many of these chemicals do other damage as well as having a carcinogenic effect. They are often directly toxic to the immune cells too – breaking down the body's first-line army or defence mechanism. Because fat is a universal solvent, many chemicals can dissolve and be stored in our fatty tissues. And this problem increases in direct proportion to how overweight we are and how little we exercise.

The mind–body connection

What is not addressed at all currently, by either conventional or environmental groups, are the effects of our mind and spirit on the body's chemistry and immune function, and on the development of cancer. Indeed, over the years much scepticism has been poured on the notion that the mind has anything whatsoever to do with physical illness. However, in the last twenty years, revolutionary developments in the field of psycho-neuroimmunology (PNI) – the study of how the mind and body are linked – have proved categorically that mind and body are inextricably connected.

We are rapidly on the way to understanding how both our state of mind and spirit and the use of mind–body techniques can profoundly affect our body's ability to resist and recover from illness. When people have become dispirited or crushed, or have lost their way in life, all medicine becomes much less effective. Conversely, when they become excited and motivated, living purposeful lives over which they feel they have control, the incidence of serious disease falls and treatment outcomes improve greatly where illness does exist. There is hard scientific data on the role of stress, depression, isolation and emotional repression in depressing our immune function, and on how these things affect our ability to both resist and ultimately survive serious disease. There is also a wealth of evidence on the role of mind–body techniques and psychological support in improving symptoms, well-being and survival rates.

However, a great deal more work needs to be done on the role of stress and distress in decreasing immunocompetence and disease resistance in the West. Such studies will be particularly important in helping to identify those at increased risk of stress-induced illness. This is because early work shows that some people have a much stronger physical response to stress and unhappiness than others. Just as there are individuals who are more vulnerable to carcinogenic chemicals, as a result of pharmacogenetic polymorphisms, it is likely that there are also people whose genetic make-up makes them more susceptible to the mind–body effects of stress, distress and isolation. Currently the jury is out on this subject. Initially it is important for us to look in more detail at the proven causes of cancer, then to examine the environmental arguments before, finally, we explore this more controversial area of the role of mind and spirit in cancer causation. So let us turn first to the number one cause of cancer – our diet.

Diet

Unhealthy diet causes 35 per cent of cancer deaths.

Western diet is currently thought to be the single most significant cause of cancer deaths in developed countries. This is a great shock to most people who tend to believe that smoking and environmental pollution are the biggest causes of cancer. Even those who have realized the important connection between diet and cancer seem to think that the cancer-causing element in our diet is food additives or environmental pollution. The current conventional wisdom, however, is that food additives and pollution are the cause in only a tiny proportion of cancer deaths. This means that it is the ratio of the different elements of fat, sugar, salt, protein, vegetables, fruit and starch in our diet which is at fault.

Diet is a proven cause of:	Diet is a likely contributory factor in:

Colon cancer
Rectal cancer
Adenomatous polyps
  (pre-cancerous tumours)
  of colon and rectum
	Breast cancer
	Prostate cancer
	Gastric (stomach) cancer
	Oesophageal (gullet) cancer
	Pancreatic cancer
	Uterine cancer
	Ovarian cancer
	Lung cancer
	Cervical cancer

Dietary imbalance

As evidence accumulates, the recurring finding is that it is plant materials known collectively as phytochemicals which protect us from cancer, whilst excessive protein, fat and sugar seriously increase our risk. Food processed to its refined white state is also a serious offender because the processing removes vital minerals, vitamins and the plant phytochemicals which are so crucial to the body's normal healthy cellular function. The dangers facing society can be quickly appreciated by considering the fact that children are currently estimated to get over 75 per cent of their daily calorie requirement from fizzy drinks and sweets. This is a major problem since these foods contain only 'empty calories' with virtually no nutritional value. At the same time, it is estimated that 47 per cent of children in the UK currently eat no vegetables whatsoever, other than chips! This means that while children may be getting more than enough energy and calories to continue to function and become obese, the vital nutrients required for healthy growth, immune function and intracellular protection from cancer are inexorably depleted, making their vulnerability to major degenerative diseases such as cancer very much heightened. It has also been shown that resulting vitamin and mineral deficiencies in children can impair learning ability as well as cause violent and disruptive behaviour. This means that our children are 'an accident waiting to happen'. This nutritional problem in children must be addressed as a matter of great urgency.

Obesity

As well as the nutritional compromise created by Western diet, the other important factor in the relationship between diet and cancer is obesity itself. American scientists have shown that when the Body Mass Index (your weight in kilos divided by the square of your height in metres; e.g. $70 \div 1.75^2$ = approximately 23) rises from 22 to 32, there is a 40 per cent increase in cancer incidence. It has certainly been noted that in prisoner of war camps, women who were more than 10 per cent underweight were never seen to have breast cancer at all. This finding has also been made in animal studies where underweight animals are very rarely seen to have cancer. This very clearly points towards the fact that cancer is a disease of affluence.

The cancers most strongly affected by obesity are cancers of the breast, endometrium (womb lining), colon (large bowel) and gall bladder. The exact reason why obesity is so important is not completely clear, but it is certainly true that body fat is a major source of oestrogen – especially in post-menopausal women. Many cancers are hormone sensitive, i.e. their growth is accelerated in the presence of high hormone levels.

As well as this extra hormonal influence on the body created by obesity, there is another problem connected with fat. Along with water, fat is a universal solvent. This means that body fat becomes a storage house for chemical toxins (organic rather than inorganic) which we absorb from our food or through our lungs. Organic chemicals are those based on a carbon ring structure which is found in man-made petrochemicals and plastics as well as many naturally occurring substances. This fatty storehouse for chemical pollutants then maintains high toxin levels in the body, subjecting the cells long term to unwanted chemical influences. People on a diet high in animal and plant fats are also absorbing and storing fats which the animals or plants have themselves stored over their lifetime. Humans, at the end of the food chain, therefore get the cumulative effect of this toxic build-up. If we are fat ourselves we are put at further risk, unless we consume exclusively organically farmed produce.

The reason mother's milk can carry over 200 chemical pollutants is that it is so high in fat. It is estimated that during breast feeding, babies are exposed to a level of environmental toxins forty times higher than at any time later in their life. However, even with this contamination, we must continue to breast feed our babies for the immunological benefits of mother's milk still far outweigh this relatively high-level exposure.

Foods and cooking methods which increase the risk of cancer

Foods

Looking more specifically at the elements within the diet which produce cancer, it is clear that excessive meat and animal fats put us at greater risk. Whilst high meat intake appears to increase the risk of colorectal cancer, the roles of other protein foods such as fish, chicken or dairy products are unclear. In case control studies, high intake of dietary fat has been associated with increased risk of many cancers, including breast, prostate, lung and colorectal. This association, however, has not been confirmed consistently in research. It has not been possible so far to distinguish between the effects of total, saturated, vegetable or animal fats. The inconsistencies in these findings may reflect varying biological effects of different fatty acids such as the omega-3 or omega-6 fatty acids, some of which may be beneficial and some adverse for tumour growth.

Links Between Specific Cancers and Dietary Factors	
Cancer Site	**Adverse Dietary Factors**
Breast	Total fat, omega-6 fatty acids, meat, alcohol
Colon and rectum	Total fat, meat, heterocyclic amines, alcohol (especially beer)

Stomach	Nitrates/nitrites, alcohol, salted and smoked foods
Oesophagus	Alcohol
Endometrium and ovaries	Saturated fat
Prostate	Saturated fat
Pancreas	Coffee
Bladder	Coffee
Lung	Saturated fat, meat

Cooking methods

There is evidence that char-grilling meat and fats, and superheating fats, create dangerous free radicals and carcinogenic compounds such as polycyclic aromatic hydrocarbons. There is concern for the same reason about the safety of smoked foods. Excessively salted and pickled foods also increase the risk of cancer, as do those which are preserved with saltpetre (potassium nitrate), such as salamis. A direct link has been identified between salted fish consumed in south China and a type of cancer found in the nose or throat area. There is also an increased incidence of gastric cancer in the Far East where higher levels of salt and salt-preserved foods are eaten.

Another very specific food contaminant, which is definitely implicated in liver cancer in undeveloped countries, is aflatoxin, a metabolic product of a fungus that contaminates grains stored in hot and humid conditions.

Protective factors in food

Fortunately, it is not all bad news. People who eat large amounts of fruit and vegetables halve their cancer risk.

The most consistent observation is a decrease in cancers of the lung, stomach and oesophagus, and a smaller but consistent decrease in cancers of the mouth, larynx, colon, breast, pancreas and bladder. Strangely, the same protection has not been seen in cancer of the prostate.

Cancers protected against most strongly by a healthy diet are those of the mouth, pharynx (throat), larynx (voice box), stomach, colon (large bowel) and rectum. The next most protected against are cancers of the breast, lung, prostate, endometrium (womb lining) and ovaries.

Initially, investigations into fruit and vegetables centred around the protective effects of antioxidant vitamins, particularly betacarotene and vitamin E, and the effects of fibre. Studies were started after scientists discovered that blood levels of betacarotene were higher in people who ate large amounts of fruit and vegetables, and that in these people there was also lower cancer incidence and fewer deaths from cancer. This led to the hypothesis that it was the betacarotene itself which was conveying the protection. However, subsequent research in which individuals were given betacarotene in tablet form to try to prevent cancer has proved very confusing. In some studies, smokers who took betacarotene ended up having a higher cancer risk than those who did not! Critics say these results are invalid because synthetic rather than natural betacarotene was used.

However, overall the research showed that people with high levels of betacarotene in their bloodstream at the beginning of the trial were better protected than those with low levels. It was those whose levels increased very rapidly during the course of the trial who seemed to be at increased risk of lung cancer. From this evidence, it must be deduced that it is not betacarotene alone which conveys the benefit, and work is now under way to investigate the contribution of the many families of plant chemicals (phytochemicals) which are thought to be implicated in cancer prevention.

Studies on the role of vitamin E are more promising. Results showed that 50 milligrams per day of vitamin E reduced the risk of prostate cancer by 40 per cent. It is also thought that calcium, vitamin D and folic acid may all reduce the risk of cancers of the colon and rectum. Other studies have highlighted the role of antioxidant vitamins C, E and betacarotene, and the mineral selenium in helping to prevent colon polyps from turning malignant.

The most exciting work in the last decade has been done with the phytochemicals in green leafy vegetables and broccoli, in yellow and orange vegetables such as yellow peppers and carrots, and in onions, tomatoes and soya products. Cabbages and broccoli (and other brassicas) have been found to contain a compound called indoleglycosi-nate, which protects against cancer. The yellow/orange vegetables have been found to contain a combination of factors, including many carotenoids, calcium, selenium and other micronutrients which work in concert to produce a strong anticancer effect. Tomatoes have been found to contain a substance called lycopene, and studies have shown an inverse relationship between body lycopene levels and cancers of the digestive tract and prostate. Soya products and fermented soya products such as miso have been found to contain phyto-oestrogens which block oestrogen activity in the same way as the anti-cancer drug tamoxifen. The plant chemicals – phytates, protease inhibitors, lignams, isoflavonoids and isoflavones – are all under investigation too, as they are all thought to be direct inhibitors of cancer genes. Studies with miso – fermented soya or barley – have shown it has definite cancer-protective effects. Lemons have been shown to contain another anti-cancer substance called limonene.

Other anti-cancer agents, which interfere with both initiation and promotion of cancer cells, have been found in shiitake mushrooms, kombu and kelp. Yet more phytochemicals from fruit and vegetables which are believed to help protect against cancer are plant phenols, aromatic isothiocyanates, thiocyanates, methylated flavones, coumarins, saponins, allium compounds, plant sterols, dithiolthiones, glucosinates and indoles, as well as naturally occurring plant selenium, zinc, copper, iron, calcium, manganese, potassium and magnesium salts (see Appendix 2 for a full list). Naturally occurring ascorbic acid (vitamin C) and its accompanying bioflavinoids and co-factors (now thought to be as important as the vitamin itself), tocopherols, B vitamins (including folic acid, B6 and riboflavin), retinols and carotenoids are also very important elements of fruit and vegetables which protect us from cancer. Many of these work together symbiotically to render harmless carcinogenic substances and to repair damage to DNA in a cell's nucleus, thereby preventing tumour formation.

Protease inhibitors, like those found in soy, are thought to protect cells from ionizing radioactivity from natural sources as well as from X-rays used in cancer therapy and diagnostic procedures.

Plant constituents such as the flavonoids and plant

oestrogens have been shown, in small studies, to alter the blood levels of sex hormones associated with prostate and breast cancer risk, but direct links have yet to be demonstrated. However, the ability to demonstrate a biological basis for diet–cancer associations in population studies considerably strengthens confidence that these relationships are causal. It is thought, for example, that the high levels of phyto-oestrogens in soy products give protection from breast cancer to women in Japan where the lifetime risk is only 1 in 45, compared with 1 in 10 in the West.

Fibre in the diet is thought to protect us in two ways. First, the phytates and lignans in fibre directly lower the production of free radicals within the body. High fibre levels in the diet also speed up the transit time of potential carcinogens through the bowel, thereby decreasing their absorption rate and lessening this harmful effect on the gut tissues they come in contact with. It is therefore likely that a healthy wholefood, predominantly vegetarian, diet protects against cancer by providing adequate levels of vitamins, minerals and phytochemicals in order to:

- promote healthy tissue growth and replication

- boost immune function

- deactivate dangerous free radicals and pollutants

- directly stabilize cell membranes and cell division processes

- promote DNA and RNA repair and proto-oncogene stabilization

It appears our grandmothers were right when they told us 'vegetables are good for you' – and not just for our skin and hair either! It is absolutely vital that we pay proper attention to diet, both as individuals and in society. We must all adopt a healthy diet – not only in our homes, but also in our restaurants, schools, hospitals and all other institutions – if we are to even begin to fight and win the war against cancer.

Smoking

Smoking causes 30 per cent of cancer deaths.

Current knowledge implicates smoking in no less than fourteen different cancers! Compared with non-smokers, cigarette smokers are:

- 15 times more likely to have lung cancer

- 10 times more likely to have cancer of the larynx (voice box) or pharynx (throat)

- 7 times more likely to have cancer of the oesophagus (gullet)

- 4 times more likely to have cancer of the pelvis, kidney or mouth

- 3 times more likely to have cancer of the bladder

- 2 times more likely to have cancer of the pancreas

- 1.5 times more likely to have cancer of the lip, nose, stomach, kidney and liver, and myeloid leukaemia

Pipe and cigar smoking are also important contributing factors in cancers of the mouth, pharynx (throat), oesophagus (gullet) and larynx (voice box), and pipe smoking is also linked to cancer of the lip. The risk of many of these cancers is further compounded by alcohol consumption – especially liver cancers. In 1995, Sir Richard Peto estimated that in developed countries smoking was responsible for 39 per cent of all cancer deaths in men and 15 per cent in women. Sadly the figure for women continues to increase as more women start to smoke. There is considerable variation in these male/female ratios throughout the developed countries of the world.

Percentage of deaths (in 1995) from cancer attributable to smoking		
Country	% Male	% Female
Australia	32	14
Denmark	38	22
France	38	2
Hungary	53	15
Italy	42	6
Japan	29	8
Netherlands	45	9
Russian Federation	55	6
Spain	34	0
Sweden	20	8
UK	40	20
USA	45	28

Permission to reprint granted by Sir Richard Doll

Smoking-related cancer deaths have generally increased over the last twenty years. Among men in France they have risen from 33 to 38 per cent. But in some countries they have decreased, most notably in the UK, where they have gone down from 52 per cent to 40 per cent among men. In women, however, the proportions have all increased, except in Spain where they are still immeasurably low because few women have been smoking for long enough for any substantial effect to be detected.

It has been shown beyond doubt that half of all regular smokers die prematurely from a smoking-related disease. As well as causing cancer, smoking is an important cause of heart attacks, strokes, chronic lung conditions, and circulation problems which can result in pain, gangrene and leg amputation. Smoking also causes tooth and gum problems and is a significant cause of peptic ulcers.

Despite the very well publicized dangers of cigarette smoking, roughly one in four adults in Western countries over the age of eighteen still smokes. A recent very alarming trend is that tobacco companies have begun to transfer their marketing effort to developing countries, as advertising restrictions become tighter and tighter in the West. This will result in the most dire consequences and suffering since most developing countries cannot even provide morphine for palliative care for people with cancer, let alone screening, medical treatment and hospice care.

The reason for the terrible medical consequences of smoking is that cigarette smoke is estimated to contain some forty different carcinogenic and irritant chemicals.

In addition, the heat of the cigarette smoke and the cigarette end (especially when there is no filter) can cause direct burning and irritation to the lips, throat and windpipe. This continual burning irritation can create ideal conditions for cancer to develop.

People continue to smoke because nicotine and other chemicals in cigarette smoke are highly addictive and the chemical 'buzz' smoking creates gives them temporary relief from tension and anxiety. Many people use cigarettes as a social and psychological prop to help them deal with the constant anxiety and stress they experience. To kick the habit, people often need emotional support to deal with these feelings. Even people's attempts to cut down their risk by smoking low-tar cigarettes have backfired in many cases. This is because people who smoke these cigarettes often inhale far more deeply to get the same levels of nicotine and as a result different patterns of lung cancer are now seen, with the tumour situated far deeper into the lung tissue.

Reproductive hormones

Excess hormones cause 10 per cent of cancer deaths.

The problem with reproductive hormones is that we are becoming exposed to an excess of human reproductive hormones to which we are not evolutionarily adjusted. As already mentioned in the section on dietary causes of cancer, both an excess of calories (and the obesity this causes) and the consumption of animal fats leads to unhealthily high hormone levels within the body. This means that throughout our lifetimes, we have much higher circulating levels of these hormones than our ancestors did.

In developing countries, where people have a far lower nutritional intake than is now common in developed countries, girls start their menstrual cycle later and women have multiple pregnancies followed by prolonged lactation. All three of these factors greatly reduce the risks of cancer of the breast, endometrium and ovaries. Later menstruation and the hormones associated with pregnancy and lactation reduce oestrogen activity in the body. Oestrogen is a very powerful hormone which prepares the womb lining for conception, the egg for release from the ovary, and the breast for the possibility of conception and subsequent lactation. In women who repeatedly go through the menstrual cycle without conceiving, the monthly oestrogenic stimulation of the tissues can lead to cancer development. If background levels of oestrogen in the body are already very high due to obesity and diet, the problem is compounded.

Added to this problem is the additional use of oestrogen hormones in birth control pills and hormone replacement therapy (HRT), both of which have been shown to increase the risk of cancer. The Pill and HRT increase the risk of breast cancer during the period they are actually being taken, and even the Combined Pill, which contains oestrogen and progesterone, increases the risk of breast cancer by 20 per cent. However, with the Pill this risk disappears once a woman stops taking it. At the same time, the Pill protects against cancer of the endometrium (womb lining) and ovaries by up to 50 per cent long term – and protection continues even after the woman has stopped taking it. Medical authorities argue that because the breast cancer rate is much lower in young women than in post-menopausal women, the risk of taking the Pill whilst young is acceptable and is outweighed by the future protection of the endometrium and ovaries.

With HRT, the increased risk of breast and endometrial cancer after ten to twenty-five years on the treatment is estimated at 20 per cent, and the risk remains the same five years after stopping. But it has also been shown that taking HRT reduces the risk of colon cancer by around 20 per cent.

As you can see, the hormone picture is complicated, and we are certainly not about to revert to a lifestyle in which women in the West have multiple pregnancies! The medical answer has been to suggest that women are given a synthetic oestrogen hormone blockade to protect them from high oestrogen levels, and therefore breast cancer, by use of the drug tamoxifen. In fact, there is a huge trial currently being conducted to look at the possibility of using tamoxifen on a widespread basis throughout society to help reduce breast cancer incidence and mortality. This has become a main plank of the research strategy for the big cancer charities but is a path that is strongly opposed by many women's action groups, which feel that the side-effects of tamoxifen are being grossly underplayed. The most notable concern is the increased risk by 5–10 per cent of endometrial (womb lining) cancer whilst taking tamoxifen. The medical charities' response to this is that tamoxifen's protection against breast cancer is fifty times greater than its risk to the womb lining, and that the benefits therefore outweigh the side-effects.

However, other serious side-effects of tamoxifen can be severe weight gain; diarrhoea; nausea; and skin, hair and even voice changes. As we know, obesity is a risk factor for breast cancer and so taking tamoxifen can create a vicious cycle. In my view, it would seem far more appropriate for us to grasp the nutritional nettle and begin to tackle the problem of obesity and excessive fat consumption, rather than taking this 'chemo-preventive' route with all the associated dangers. The next chapter will give clear advice for women facing these 'hormonal dilemmas'.

The medical profession has no equivalent solution for the prevention of cancer of the prostate, apart from the possible benefits of taking vitamin E. It is believed, however, that ultimately cancer of the testis will be preventable by a change in some lifestyle or environmental factor; the fact that its incidence has risen so dramatically in the latter half of the last century indicates that it must be something we are doing differently which is causing the problem.

Infection

Infection causes 10 per cent of cancer deaths.

A large number of cancers are caused worldwide by parasites, bacteria and viruses and it is likely that as our understanding increases, the assessment of the percentage risk from these agents to the cause of cancer will grow. The role of bacteria and parasites is much greater in developing countries, whereas the role of the virus is more ubiquitous. In Africa and Asia, many cancers of the bladder, colon (large bowel), liver and bile ducts are caused by parasite infections, all of which could be avoided with a combination of environmental and therapeutic measures. These parasites play little or no role in cancer causation in developed countries.

The role of bacteria in causing cancer of the stomach and digestive tract has received much attention recently, but latterly the role of bacteria in cancer of the large bowel has been questioned. The theory was that gut bacteria may turn bile salts into carcinogens, but at present this theory is looking less likely. On the other hand, the recently discovered *Helicobacter pylori* bacterium has been shown to significantly contribute to cancer of the stomach, as well as to stomach ulcers. However, this is not a straightforward relationship because, in other countries where the incidence of helicobacter is high, there is a low incidence of cancer of the stomach. Even more confusing is the finding that where helicobacter is eradicated through antibiotics used to treat gastric ulcers, the incidence of oesophageal and lung cancer increases!

It is possible that chronic bacterial infection of the bladder may be a cause of bladder cancer because the bacteria can produce waste products (called nitrosamines) which are carcinogenic and over time may cause the disease.

Viruses are a much bigger and more serious cause of cancer altogether, responsible for the great majority of two of the most common cancers worldwide – of the liver and the cervix. They are also involved in many of the less common cancers. Strangely, the viruses listed below are not associated with every case of the cancers they can cause. Also, it is often found that compounding factors need to be involved before the viruses cause a problem. For example, the virus which causes Burkitt's lymphoma in Africa has its effect in the presence of malarial parasites, and in many cases the virus causing liver cancer has its effect in the presence of aflatoxin.

Viral Causes of Cancer	
Virus	**Cancer**
Hepatitis B	Hepatocarcinoma
Hepatitis C	Hepatocarcinoma
Human papillomavirus (HPV), types 16, 18 and others	Cancer of the cervix, vulva, vagina, penis and anus
Human herpes type 4 (Epstein-Barr virus)	Lymphoma, immunoblastic lymphoma, nasal T-cell lymphoma, Hodgkin's disease, naso-pharyngeal cancer
Human herpes type 8	Kaposi's sarcoma
(Kaposi's associated herpes virus)	Body cavity lymphoma
Human T-cell leukaemia type 1	Adult T-cell leukaemia/lymphoma
Simian virus 40-like	Ependymoma, choroid plexus tumours, mesothelioma and bone tumours
Herpes simplex type II (genital herpes)	Cancer of the vagina, penis and anus
Human immunodeficiency virus (HIV)	Lymphoma
Acquired immune deficiency syndrome (AIDS)	Kaposi's sarcoma

Permission to reprint granted by Sir Richard Doll

HPV, HIV and the herpes viruses can all be transmitted sexually (as can hepatitis C on rare occasions). The practice of safe sex has therefore far wider importance than the public currently realize. We have been given a very strong message about safe sex in relation to HIV, but the message is much less strong in relation to HPV, which is an important cause of cervical cancer and premature death in women.

The medical profession is concentrating its efforts on the role of vaccinations in preventing these virally triggered cancers. It is already possible to immunize against hepatitis, and widespread immunization is being introduced in some tropical and semitropical countries where hepatitis infection is more common than in developed countries. It is hoped the HPV vaccine will be available to women within ten years, in particular to help prevent cervical cancer.

It is certainly my hunch that viruses set the scene for many more of the common cancers than we currently realize. Viruses transmitted through the animal food chain may yet turn out to be the real reason why the eating of meat and other animal products is so strongly implicated in raised cancer risk.

Alcohol

Alcohol causes 5 per cent of cancer deaths.

Alcohol is estimated to cause an average of 5 per cent of cancer deaths in developed countries, but the rates can vary from 3 to as much as 12 per cent in different countries. Heavy alcohol drinkers are:

- 3 times more likely to have cancer of the oesophagus (gullet) than non-drinkers

- 2 times more likely to have cancers of the mouth, pharynx (throat) and larynx (voice box)

- 1.5 times more likely to have cancer of the liver

- 1.2 times more likely to have breast cancer.

The role of alcohol in the development of breast cancer is the most recent discovery of all these associations. It is thought that this effect is caused by alcohol's ability to raise hormone levels in the body. Evidence gathered in 1993 by Reichmann (showing that alcohol increased the level of oestrogens in the blood) put the causal relationship between alcohol and breast cancer beyond reasonable doubt. These risks have been assessed on the basis of an 'average consumption' of alcohol. The risk increases in heavy drinkers. The high-risk levels associated with cancers of the mouth, throat, gullet and voice box are all significantly lower in non-smokers.

The message for us all is to reduce our drinking dramatically – you can still have a glass of wine or beer, but stick within the safe limits of two units a day for women, three for men. In fact, other evidence shows a small amount of alcohol (one glass of wine per day) can reduce the risk of heart attack. Some people argue that this is a good reason to continue a low level of alcohol consumption. However, it is likely that this cardiovascular protection is caused by the relaxing effect of alcohol and the nutritional benefits of the vitamins and minerals in wine. These effects can easily be achieved in safer ways, through self-help practices such as yoga, meditation, relaxation and a healthy diet, without any of alcohol's toxicity to the body, so don't feel you have to drink to stay healthy!

Anyone who has ever drunk too much or suffered a hangover can be under no illusion whatsoever about the toxicity of alcohol. Its role in degenerative disease of many kinds has been proved beyond any shadow of doubt. The liver, gut, mental health, social and cancer problems alcohol creates make it public enemy number two after smoking. If alcohol were introduced now as a new drug it would probably be judged a Class A illegal substance because of the profound risks associated with its use. Unfortunately, alcohol use is so deeply embedded within Western culture as our major recreational drug that any governmental attempt to control its consumption would probably result in civil war! So once again, it comes down to the role of the individual in changing behaviour patterns if there is to be any improvement in alcohol-related cancer statistics.

For many people changing their use of alcohol represents an even more serious challenge than giving up smoking, and addressing this challenge will be given very serious consideration in the next chapter. Certainly, of the two, the priority is to give up smoking because this will at least reduce the risk of lung cancer as well as decrease the risk to the windpipe and gullet posed by alcohol.

Electromagnetic radiation

EMR causes 4 per cent of cancer deaths.

In developed countries, ultraviolet radiation from sunlight is responsible for most melanomas and nearly all squamous and basal cell cancers of the skin. Added to this is the effect of naturally occurring radioactivity or background radioactivity, which is produced naturally by radon and its decay products in the earth.

Radioactivity

Radon is estimated to account for around 6 per cent of all lung cancers in the UK and as many as 18 per cent in France. Again, the effects of radon and smoking act synergistically, and stopping smoking makes radon exposure far less dangerous. As far as natural sources of radioactivity go, it is possible to ascertain from local environmental agencies the radon levels in your area, and if you are concerned your home can be checked for radon gas.

There is also widespread concern about the effects of radioactive leakage and contamination from nuclear power stations and nuclear waste dumping. Controversy continues about the roles of nuclear power stations in cancer causation, but certainly clusters of childhood leukaemia have been seen around power stations. It is possible that power station workers and local people are being affected by radioactive contamination, and that these effects are being passed on to their offspring through affected sperm or eggs.

The ethics of nuclear power remain, in my opinion,

highly questionable. It seems irresponsible to create more and more radioactive material and waste material which as yet cannot be eliminated and which has to buried or dumped in the sea where it will remain radioactive for extremely long periods. To leave this ghastly legacy for future generations for thousands of years to come is an appalling crime against humanity and nature and it seems very wrong that it is legal to do so.

Certainly nuclear accidents and exposure to radioactive materials of any sort are associated with very marked increases in cancer incidence. After the Chernobyl disaster, levels of thyroid cancer in the region rose dramatically due to the spillage of radioactive iodine which then became concentrated in the thyroid glands of people living within a considerable radius of the site. The main cause of death in those who are not killed outright by a nuclear explosion is cancer, which can go on appearing for years after the original blast.

Medical X-rays are also a source of considerable concern. It has been shown that X-rays to the mother's abdomen during pregnancy cause 5 per cent of leukaemias in children.

Individually, we must take the utmost care to ensure that, if possible, we are not living or working close to sources of radiation – either natural radioactivity from the earth in the form of radon, or the man-made variety in military weapons, chemical factories, power stations or nuclear dumps. People who do work or live near sources of radiation must be very vigilant and keep in close touch with local authorities for constant information and reassurance about levels of radioactivity in the area and the proper implementation of safety measures.

Unproven, but of concern, is the effect of radiation emitted from computer screens on our brains and immune systems. There is some evidence of increased incidence of brain tumours, leukaemias and lymphomas in those who are stuck in front of computers day after day. The general advice for people who spend long hours in front of a computer is to use screens to help defuse the radiation emitted and take regular screen breaks.

Ultraviolet radiation

Atmospheric pollution has played a serious role in increasing our risk of skin cancer. The three main skin cancers – melanoma, squamous and basal cell cancer – are all caused by over exposure to UV light. Normally, the ozone layer mops up the majority of ultraviolet light from the sun. But, because of the damage to the ozone layer and the resulting hole which has been created by CFCs from fridges and aerosols, people are being exposed to far higher levels of ultraviolet radiation than normal. Certainly this has had an adverse effect on skin cancer incidence in Australia, which has been particularly badly affected.

Ultraviolet light is made up of UVA, UVB and UVC rays. Usually, only a small amount of UVA and UVB reaches the earth. It is the UVB rays which burn our skin and are probably the most important cancer-producing agent. But, in recent years, experimental studies in animals have suggested that UVA rays penetrate the skin layer more deeply than UVB rays (without burning it) and may also play an important role in cancer development. Individuals with pale skin or freckles, blue eyes, red or fair hair and who burn easily in the sun, are more prone to skin damage than those with olive or dark skins, and should be particularly careful.

It is also important to remember that UVA rays from sunbeds can potentially overstimulate our skin. These beds have been declared safe by medical authorities but, as with so many things, it is all a matter of degree. There is also the question of whether the machine is working according to manufacturers' specifications.

Cancer research charities go as far as saying that there is no such thing as a healthy tan. Their advice is to avoid getting a suntan altogether, and to wear sun block and protective clothing when in hot countries. If a tanned look is desired, their advice would therefore be to avoid the use of sunbeds and opt instead for tanning milks which stain the skin.

Electricity

Another source of concern is the possible link between cancer and electromagnetic radiation from pylons, wires, high-voltage units and electrical household equipment. Recently a correlation has been found between extra-low-frequency electric fields and the incidence of childhood leukaemia and male breast cancer. There is also an observed risk of brain tumours in electric power company workers.

In the past, it has been hard to prove any connection between the electromagnetic fields of high-voltage electrical equipment and cancer. But recent work in Bristol has shown that in some situations it may not be the electromagnetic field itself which is creating a hazard, but radioactive particles that are attracted into the field. It is unwise to live and work close to high-voltage electrical equipment of any sort or to live over buried electrical cabling.

In general, our environments are becoming more and more electrical and it is not unusual to work in buildings with many hundreds of computer terminals surrounded by layer upon layer of electrical cabling within the walls. If you are concerned it is possible to get your employer, the local electricity board or the Department of the Environment to measure the electromagnetic fields in offices or shops with highly electrical environments, or in your home if you live close to high-voltage terminals and pylons.

Radiowaves and microwaves
In addition to being surrounded by electrical fields, we are being bombarded by radiowaves and microwaves from ever-increasing broadcasting and the rapidly rising use of mobile phones. There is much concern about the microwave emanations from mobile phones themselves and their possible link with brain cancer. Currently, medical authorities feel the risk is small but the picture is still far from clear.

There are also questions about the effects of the many radio and telephone masts which are being erected throughout cities and the countryside and the role of the radio- and microwaves on our genetic material. It is clear that, once again, the commercial sector is racing ahead of the scientists and that currently the telecommunications industry has not fully researched the potential risks of the equipment they are installing and selling.

Microwave ovens are another source of potential risk

if they are used improperly or if they are faulty and directly expose the user to microwaves. Microwaved food may itself cause trauma to the mouth, oesophagus (gullet) and stomach if proper standing times are not observed. Microwave energy is a very-high-frequency energy, which heats food very rapidly to temperatures beyond those reached by normal cooking methods. Whilst this is very questionable nutritionally – because vitamins and vital plant enzymes and phytochemicals are destroyed at high temperatures – it is also very probable that if the intense microwave radiation is not allowed to dissipate properly before the food is eaten, it can cause burning and tissue damage to the digestive tract. Repeated irritation to the mucous membrane in this way could easily be a cause of future cancer.

Clearly there is still a great deal we do not know about microwave technology, and until the science is clearer, great care should be taken in the use of mobile phones and microwave ovens.

Sound

Another little-researched and little-understood subject is the effect of sound on the body. At certain frequencies sound can have both very beneficial and very damaging effects on human tissue. There has been concern about the use of ultrasound in medical practice and whether this is a cause of cancer. I also question the effect of sound in modern clubs where young people are bombarded with increasingly loud and chaotic noise. Some clubs are even placing speakers under the floor as well as on the walls in order to send intense vibration energy through the feet of the dancers whilst they are listening to the music, though, in fact, the vibrations they feel through the floor are slightly out of phase with what they are hearing. Again, these practices are being employed without any knowledge as to the potential damage which could be created by subjecting the body to these intense chaotic vibrational patterns.

Earth energies
More controversial is the question of the earth's electro-magnetic field and the role of the currents created by the underlying rock formation. The 'earth energies' and 'lay lines' created have been implicated in the development of cancer. Studies by dowsers who can track these currents have shown very specific clusters of cancer along the lay lines in cities which have been fully mapped. This is an area which has as yet received no serious scientific study, but is one which should be looked into by individuals and cancer researchers for the correlations are too high to be ignored. It may well be that a strange underlying phe-nomenon like this will solve the mystery of the often seem-ingly random nature of cancer distribution among people who are all broadly exposed to the same risk factors.

Environmental pollution

Pollution causes 2.5 per cent of cancer deaths.

Public concern about environmental pollution and cancer is very high, although medical authorities estimate it to cause only 2 per cent of cancer deaths. The main areas of concern are:

- industrial waste
- pollution of the air with diesel and petrol fumes and the products of waste (particularly plastic) combustion
- the by-products of intensive agriculture
- chemicals used at home, in food additives and in building, cleaning, DIY and gardening products

Asbestos

Asbestos, which was used extensively in building during the twentieth century for roofing, insulation and as part of floor tiles, is one very specific substance which has been proved beyond doubt to be associated with cancer of the lining of the lung (mesothelioma). Unfortunately, asbestos fibres crumble easily and minute particles which can only be seen under a microscope get into the air and become inhaled deeply into the lung tissue or swallowed. These particles can lodge in the throat and lungs, and sometimes go down into the gut, causing damage in the stomach and bowel, in some cases leading to cancer. As well as causing mesothelioma, asbestos has been implicated in cancer of the larynx (voice box) and also possibly of the oesophagus (gullet), stomach and ovaries. The worst kinds of asbestos are the blue and brown varieties. The white kind is less dangerous because the body is more able to eliminate it.

There are now very strict guidelines for the use and removal of asbestos from buildings and it is most unwise for untrained individuals to deal with any asbestos fibre problem in the home, whatever type of asbestos involved. If there is any concern about the presence of asbestos – for example, it may have become damaged through age – it is vital to obtain the help of experts who are certified by the local environmental agencies to advise on its removal.

Persistent chemicals

Great concern has developed about the effect of industrial, transport, waste disposal and farming pollution because of the dangerous persistent chemicals they leave in the environment. Environmentalists have reported cancers in fish linked to the pollution of lakes with polycyclic aromatic hydrocarbons found in petroleum products, and mass sterility amongst wildlife. This, combined with falling sperm levels in human males, has triggered widespread anxiety about the cancer risk to humans from environmental carcinogens and about tumour promotion by hormonally active pollutants known as endocrine disrupters.

A Danish study found that the average male sperm count dropped by 45 per cent between 1940 and 1990. The volume of the semen ejaculated had also dropped by 25 per cent, making an effective sperm decline of 50 per cent. There has also been a big increase in the rates of testicular cancer among young men during the same period. Exposure of male babies in the womb to elevated oestrogen levels (from diet and chemical oestrogens in the environment) may increase the risk of testicular tumours, prostate cancer and benign prostatic disease in later life.

Environmental campaigners have homed in on the possible role of hormone-mimicking organochlorine pesticides in the development of cancer. Past and current use of organochlorine pesticides has led to pollution of the entire globe, with detectable levels in the body fat of nearly everyone worldwide. Of particular concern has been the question of whether organochlorine pesticides are one of the environmental factors responsible for the rise in breast cancer, because of their oestrogen-mimicking activity. The persistence of these chemicals in the environment, and their accumulation in animals at the top of the food chain, has led to the introduction of measures to control their use. In the UK many organochlorine pesticides – including DDT, aldrin, chlordane, dieldrin, heptachlor and toxaphene – have been banned, but DDT and others are still widely used in many parts of the world. The organochlorine pesticide lindane is still currently approved for use in the UK.

Packaging, particularly plastic, is another source of hormone-disrupting chemicals. They may also be found in ointments, cosmetics, shampoos and other common household products. A large number of man-made chemicals (as well as a few natural ones) which have been released into the environment have the potential to disrupt the hormone system of animals, including humans. Among these are the persistent bio-accumulative organohalogen compounds found in some pesticides, fungicides, herbicides, insecticides, industrial chemicals, other synthetic products and some metals.

Examples of those chemicals in the environment known to disrupt the endocrine system can be found in

Appendix 2. If they find their way into the body, many of these compounds imitate the action of oestrogen. Unless the environmental load of synthetic hormone or endocrine disrupters is abated and controlled, large-scale problems in the population are possible. In studies on rats, organochlorine compounds have been shown to promote already-existing breast tumours, although none of the pesticides actually triggered the breast cancer. The argument against these chemicals is weakened, however, by the fact that, in reality, most people have been exposed to fairly minuscule amounts of organochlorine pesticides through food, and levels in body tissues in the UK are low and have been falling.

Several studies have compared pesticide levels in women with breast cancer to levels in women without the disease. In a New York study, women with the highest blood levels of DDE (a breakdown product of DDT) were four times more likely to develop breast cancer than women with the lowest levels. Similar but not significant trends were found in three other case controlled studies. However, in a much larger study of 300 women – half of whom had breast cancer – there was no significant relation between DDE levels and the disease. Taking all the research and arguments into account, the evidence that organochlorine pesticides increase the risk of breast cancer is fairly weak. However, we must continue to strive vigorously towards organic farming for many other ecological and health reasons, most particularly to raise the nutritional quality of our food.

Agricultural practices

Another source of potential pollution are agricultural processes which contribute to nitrate contamination of food and water. These include the ploughing up of grassland for arable farming (the grass leaks nitrates into the soil), the excessive use of mineral fertilizers, poor management of slurry from animal husbandry, and inappropriate use of organic fertilizer. The problem arises when nitrates are converted to nitrosamines in the body, for most nitrosamines which have been tested are carcinogenic in animals. Within the body, the antioxidant vitamins C and E prevent nitrosamines from forming.

Certain types of vegetables such as spinach and lettuce are nitrophilic – that is, they accumulate more nitrates from the soil than they can convert into protein. Organically grown nitrophilic vegetables are less contaminated with nitrates than conventional vegetables. This is another argument for choosing organic vegetables.

However, because increased vegetable consumption provides the body with a rich source of antioxidants, the net effect is that high vegetable consumption protects against digestive tract cancers regardless of the presence of nitrates in the vegetables and the presence of pesticides and fertilizers. There is no real support from studies that nitrates in vegetables cause cancer, and there are inconsistent results demonstrating an association between cancer and nitrates in drinking water. And so, again, evidence about the possible role of nitrates in the development of cancer is weak and conflicting.

Another area of concern within intensive farming is the use of growth promoters in animal husbandry. In the past, these chemicals – a mixed bag of hormones, antibiotics, beta-agonists and copper, among others – have been used to increase milk and meat production. Of these, the one chemical which could be potentially linked to cancer is growth hormone. These substances are now banned in most developed countries and routine surveillance does not show widespread illegal use. There does not, therefore, appear to be much cause for concern about widespread exposure to these hormones in the developed parts of the world, but steps must be taken to ensure that their use is not adopted in developing countries. Whilst there are many other health concerns, there is no obvious mechanism by which antibiotics or copper used as feed additives could contribute to cancer.

Conventional wisdom suggests that animal hormones in the meat and dairy products we eat do not have biological activity in the human body. However, once again it may be a matter of degree. For those people with a diet heavily orientated towards animal foods, with high levels of butter, cream, cheese, milk and meat, the intake of animal hormones may compound the hormone-raising effects of obesity which this type of diet almost always causes.

Genetic modification
The possible relationship between the production of genetically modified crops and future cancer is a very topical question. The whole subject of genetic modification is intensely emotive because changing genetic material is the starting point of the whole cancer process. Even with the natural built-in levels of protection against

genetic mutation within the body, our genetic material is highly vulnerable in today's world, as the soaring rates of cancer show. To introduce another element of disruption into the genetic blueprint of nature would seem, potentially, to be pouring fuel on the fire, inviting genetic catastrophe in the future.

It is always reckless to introduce significant scientific or technological change before the repercussions are fully understood. In the realms of both genetics and technology, we are seeing development which is far outstripping our ability to foresee where this evolutionary path will take us, let alone the profound consequences it may have for nature and mankind. I therefore feel that if we wish to protect ourselves from cancer long term we should be extremely cautious about genetic modification and stick to working with nature rather than trying to modify it.

Regulation and taking action

Even though the cancer threat from environmental pollution is currently thought to be relatively small, we must not be complacent. The environmental situation may well have a bearing on the cancer risk associated with food and infection, and certainly the effects of sunlight are worsened by the results of pollution on the ozone layer. The situation is also worsening daily as traffic pollution increases and hundreds, possibly thousands, of new synthetic chemicals go onto the market each year, faster than toxicologists and regulatory agencies are able to develop new ways to detect and check them. Theo Colburn states in her impressive book *Our Stolen Future*, an investigation into the effect of industrial pollution on wild life and human health, 'What is happening to the animals in Florida, English rivers, the Baltic, the High Arctic, the Great Lakes and Lake Baikal in Siberia has immediate relevance to humans. The damage seen in wildlife has ominously foreshadowed symptoms that appear to be increasing in the human population. Humans and animals share the common environment as well as the common genetic evolutionary legacy. Living in a man-made landscape we easily forget that our well-being is rooted in natural systems yet all human enterprise rests on the foundation of natural systems, that provide a myriad of invisible life support services. Our connections to these natural systems may be less direct and obvious than those of an eagle or an otter but we are no less deeply implicated in life's web.'

Whilst the contribution of environmental pollution to cancer appears small, a great deal is still unknown and constant vigilance is necessary. It is absolutely crucial that we all develop a sense of the sacredness of our environment, and take action to protect it both by doing our bit at home and by setting up green initiatives in our places of work and communities. It is imperative that anyone wishing to prevent cancer, personally or collectively, becomes involved in and actively supports the environmental charities and continues to lobby their local council and all political parties to ensure that they keep the protection of the environment at the very top of their agenda.

The home environment
As our homes are the places where we spend the majority of our time, it is particularly important to think about our exposure to cancer-causing chemicals (carcinogens) there.

The main risks in the home are:

- passive smoking (the intake of cigarette, pipe or tobacco smoke from other family members, or guests)

- chemicals found in cleaners, solvents, pesticides and cosmetics, and in products used in DIY, decorating and hobbies

Increasingly, the potential risk of cancer from many other household products and cosmetics whose use we take for granted is being brought to our attention.

Household carcinogens

Household products which can contain carcinogens include:

Disinfectants, all-purpose cleaners, bathroom cleaner, scouring powder, furniture polishes, metal polishes, home dry-cleaning spot removers, toilet bowl cleaners and deodorizers, paints, varnishes, paint removers and strippers, home and garden pesticides, cat litter, flea collars and flea and tick products, interior and exterior cleaners and protectants, car waxes, art and craft supplies, typing correction fluids, glues, moth repellent, shoe polishes, cosmetics, hair dye, sunscreens, colourings, synthetic fragrances, dandruff shampoos, hairsprays, mouthwashes, toothpastes and powders, feminine care body powders, bubble baths and shaving creams. There is also a slight cancer risk associated with the use of electric blankets and with exposure to electrical goods and wiring which cause low-frequency electromagnetic fields.

Not all brands of the above products contain carcinogenic chemicals; to check definitively consult *The Safe Shopper's Bible* by David Steinman and Samuel Epstein (see Appendix 1). These authors have made a comprehensive assessment of the chemical contents of almost all Western brands of household goods and have been brave enough to publish it, showing exactly which brands present a potential risk of cancer, hormonal effects, neurotoxicity and other acute medical problems. A comprehensive list of the offending chemicals to check for can be found in Appendix 2. Be aware that nitrites, which can cause problems in the presence of other chemicals, are often undisclosed or go under the heading of 'preservatives'.

In general, for non-toxic cleaning, both for people and the environment, Steinman and Epstein recommend the use of:

Baking soda	as an excellent cleaner and deodorizer
Beeswax	for polishing
Borax	as a disinfectant
Distilled white vinegar	as an excellent cleaner
Essential oils	to add natural fragrances to home-made cleaning products
Hydrogen peroxide	as a bleach
Lemon juice	as an excellent cleaner
Liquid soap	as an alternative to harsher detergents and cleaning agents

Pumice stone	as a stain remover
Sodium perborate	as an alternative to bleaches made with sodium hypo-chlorite
Sodium percarbonate	as above
Trisodium phosphate (TSP)	as a powerful cleaning agent
Washing soda (sodium carbonate)	as a strong cleaner
Zeolite	as an excellent deodorizer

Occupational exposure

Occupational hazards cause 2 per cent of cancer deaths.

The number of occupations in which there is an increased risk of cancer is extensive and there is a long list of likely or known cancer-producing agents in the workplace (see Appendix 2).

Earlier last century, it was estimated that one in twenty-five cancers had a major occupational component but now, with strict control measures in the workplace enforced over the past generation, it is estimated that the number of work-related cancers has halved, at least in developed countries. The key issue for individuals is to know exactly what carcinogenic chemicals are used at their place of work and how they should be handled. The recom-mended protective clothing should be worn at all times. It is particularly important to find out and observe the rules if you are self-employed. The biggest offenders in this area are likely to be artists, builders and farmers, who can put themselves at serious risk if they fail to protect themselves properly from the chemicals they are using.

Physical inactivity

Physical inactivity causes 1.5 per cent of cancer deaths.

As long ago as 1912, an Englishman called the Honorable Rollo Russell said in a book on the preventable causes of cancer that 'sedentary occupations are highly injurious for cancer'. In the 1980s, men with sedentary occupations were found to be more prone to cancer of the colon. This link prompted further research into the role of exercise in the development of cancer in general. Physical inactivity is now linked to colon, breast, testicular, ovarian and prostate cancers and to colon adenoma (which can be pre-cancerous). Exercise may reduce the risk of certain cancers by:

- decreasing total body fat
- stimulating immune function
- favourably affecting hormonal balance
- speeding up large bowel transit time (the time it takes for food to pass through the gut)

Certainly in the Oriental model of health and disease, all illness is seen as being related to the stagnation of *chi* or 'vital energy' in the human body. It has been clearly stated that critical damage to genetic material occurs in toxic cellular environments when the concentration of disrupting chemicals reaches a certain level. Exercise is the best way of regularly flushing toxins out of the body, and it comes as no surprise that cancer rates are favourably affected by exercise.

Blood is pumped by the heart through the arteries into the tissues of the body. But when tissue fluids make their way back to the heart through the veins and lymph vessels, there is no pump mechanism other than the muscular movements of the body. As muscles contract during exercise such as walking, bending or stretching, the tissues are literally 'milked', causing the tissue fluid containing toxins to re-enter the lymph vessels and veins. From there, toxins are taken to the liver and kidneys to be broken down and eliminated from the body.

This muscular pumping action also helps to bring toxins to the surface of the body where they are excreted through the skin. You may well have noticed the way sweat can smell of curry the day after eating Indian food, or that the sweat of meat-eaters is far more pungent than that of vegetarians. These examples show how important skin is as a route of excretion. Concern has been expressed about the possible role of underarm deodorants in the development of cancer, because many contain strong antiperspirants which literally block excretion through the skin under the arm. This could, theoretically, result in an accumulation of toxic material in (particularly breast) tissue after prolonged use. But currently, conventional wisdom is that this does not constitute a serious health risk.

The lungs also get rid of toxins, by literally exhaling them. For example, after garlic is eaten, the aroma of garlic on the breath is very noticeable. Many people think the smell comes from the mouth or stomach but it actually comes directly from the lungs, in the breath. Excretion of toxins via the lungs increases with exercise, as the breathing rate and depth increases.

When people do not exercise, these vital processes of elimination become severely compromised. I believe that physical inactivity as a cause of cancer may still be underestimated. Certainly, it is likely to play a significant role as people grow older. Until recently, it was not unusual for people with Western lifestyles over the age of thirty to take no exercise at all apart from the occasional walk. But fortunately this trend has changed over the past thirty years. The recognition of the importance of exercise in preventing heart disease gave sport and exercise a big boost, resulting in the jogging craze of the 1970s and 1980s. However, since then, general emphasis on the 'body beautiful' has led to a wholesale return of people of all age groups to the gym and dance classes in pursuit of both the perfect physique and the greatly improved well-being and vitality which accompanies serious exercise.

Another interesting observation is that there is more cancer of the left breast than the right. As the majority of women are right handed, it stands to reason that the right arm and breast are being moved and exercised more than the left. Indeed many women hold a great deal of tension in their left shoulder and arm, holding the left arm closer to the body than the right one, effectively limiting the flow of blood and lymph under the left arm. For this reason it is a good idea to check regularly for tension in the left arm and shoulder (or right if you are left handed) and also to stretch your arms up above your head several times a day.

There is even scientific evidence that wearing a bra increases the risk of breast cancer. One of the early signs of breast cancer, which can be seen on a CT or ultrasound scan, is the presence of calcium deposits within the breast tissue. This occurs where the tissue becomes 'stagnant' (in Chinese terms), allowing the build-up of these chalky deposits. When a woman is wearing a bra, especially an under-wired one, there is less movement of the breast and it is thought that this slows down the toxin-clearing process from the breast. Breast cancer incidence increases with both larger breast size and the wearing of bras, and it is thought that this may have muddled the research findings. More research is therefore needed before definitive advice can be given about the safety of bras.

Medical procedures

Medical procedures cause 0.5 per cent of cancer deaths.

It is disturbing to learn that medical procedures can themselves be a cause of cancer deaths. Paradoxically, all the treatments for cancer are themselves carcinogenic. Quite frequently, if a person with cancer is fortunate enough to survive the disease, a second quite different cancer can develop in another part of the body because of the carcinogenic effects of chemo- and radiotherapy. In this situation the new cancer is not a secondary of the old one, but a different cancer altogether which has been triggered by the treatments. For example, tamoxifen, the oestrogen-blocking drug commonly used to help improve the prognosis of breast cancer, carries a 5–10 per cent risk of causing endometrial (womb lining) cancer.

Birth control pills and hormone replacement therapy increase the risk of cancer, and repeated X-rays, CT and magnetic resonance scans, and possibly ultrasound scans, are also linked to the development of the disease. All of these tests involve exposing the body to electromagnetic radiation, which at high levels can cause cancer – particularly in susceptible individuals. As mentioned previously, abdominal X-rays of pregnant women are estimated to cause 5 per cent of childhood leukaemia.

Obviously, great care must be taken to keep medical radiation exposure within safe limits. But it is difficult to be sure what the safe limit is for a given patient, especially when confounding factors such as occupational exposure, poor diet, smoking or a genetic predisposition exist.

Cancerous tumours are also more likely to develop in people on immunosuppressive drugs, which are required after organ transplantation. Typically, these patients are more likely to develop lymphoma. There are other rarer cancers too, which can be triggered by medical procedures, drugs and tests.

The fact that modern medicine can cause cancer is a very good incentive to try to prevent disease, and it is advisable to avoid medical testing and drugs unless they are absolutely necessary and as safe as possible. Most major hospitals now have Drug Information Centres which are open to the general public. Your doctor may not have the time to go into the possible side-effects of all the drugs, tests and treatments you are being offered, so it is well worth talking to the drug information team or the staff of the radiology department to find out the relevant detail prior to embarking on treatments or medical tests.

Cancer and the Mind

The notion that state of mind is somehow linked to the chance of getting cancer has been around for centuries. In the second century AD, the Greek physician Galen said that 'melancholic women are more prone to cancer than sanguine women'. In 1800, an eminent doctor called Walshe pointed to 'the influence of mental misery, sudden reverse of fortune and habitual gloomings of temper on the disposition of carcinomatous matter'. And in 1870, Paget noted that 'deep mental distress is among the conditions favourable to the occurrence of cancer'. During the mid-1900s, the concept of a 'cancer personality' emerged.

People thought to be especially prone to cancer were those who were unable to express hostile feelings, had a rigid personality and a tendency towards social conformity (doing what was expected of them by society), lacked self-awareness, had a tendency towards introspection, self-blame and feelings of hopelessness and despair, and were likely to have few outlets for their emotions.

Psychologist Lawrence LeShan refined this concept in the 1960s and 1970s. He found that the lives of people who get cancer are marked by feelings of isolation, neglect and despair during childhood, followed by relationship problems and the development of a consuming interest (either in a strong and meaningful relationship or a satisfying vocation) which becomes the centre of their life as an adult. Loss of this relationship or role results in despair, reactivating the painful feelings of childhood.

LeShan found that these people were also more likely to bottle up despair and be 'kind, sweet and benign' while hiding feelings of anger, hurt and hostility.

Over time, the same themes have kept recurring, with the strong suggestion that stress, bottled-up emotions, traumatic life events, isolation and depression are linked to cancer, or certainly to a worse prognosis in cancer.

However, during the late 1980s and 1990s, conventional scientific research into the role of stress and life events on cancer has been conflicting. While some studies have shown positive associations, others have not. But we should not be too quick to discount a theory that has been around for so long. It seems very likely that it will be shown that it is not stress as such that affects physical health but how well or badly different individuals cope with it.

When considering psychological influences on cancer, several factors need to be taken into account. First, cancer rates are higher, and sufferers die sooner, if they are isolated, depressed or socially disadvantaged. Of course, there are many aspects of being socially disadvantaged, such as poor nutrition, which could lead to an increased risk of cancer. But it is also very common indeed that socially dis-advantaged people are disempowered, unexpressed cre-atively, feeling frustrated and depressed as a result.

Second, there was strong evidence from the eminent psycho-social oncologist Dr Stephen Greer in the 1980s that people with cancer who have a strong 'fighting spirit' survive much longer with the same cancer than those who become 'helpless and hopeless'. Other studies have shown that patients who receive help to express their negative feelings in a support group also survive longer. These groups help patients to express their anger, grief, fear and despair, and this act of emotional expression carries a very significant survival benefit.

Third, patients who practise the mind–body technique of visualization (imagining positive outcomes to treatment) whilst having chemotherapy for cancer also have better survival rates. In this technique, once patients are relaxed they are given a series of very positive images to visualize (of the benefits they should receive from their chemother-apy) whilst they are actually having the treatment. These studies also showed that people with very high social con-formity benefited particularly profoundly in terms of long term survival, having a 13 per cent improvement in sur-vival rate fifteen years after the intervention.

Fourth, on a much more anecdotal level, anyone involved in the care of people with cancer will tell you that when they lose their will to live, death can follow very quickly, no matter what medicine, orthodox or com-plementary, is being given. And there is even research from the United States which shows that difficult patients survive longer! Another interesting phenomenon is that while more women get breast cancer in the US than in the UK, fewer die of it. Medics believe this is to do with better screening or medicine in the US. But my own hunch is that it may well be due to the far more assertive, upbeat reaction of most Americans and their doctors to the diagnosis and illness management, and to lower levels of depression and far higher levels of fighting spirit. By contrast, the response to cancer diagnosis in the UK is often very passive and gloomy, with many doctors tending to crush patients' efforts to fight the disease rather than encouraging attempts at self-help.

All this evidence suggests strongly that our state of mind most definitely does affect the progress of cancer growth in the body, although it still seems highly unlikely that particular states of mind will ever be shown to be an actual cause of cancer. What does seem likely is that negative states of mind do have a direct effect on the immune system and tissue functioning, weakening the body's defences against cancer. The new field of psychoneuroimmunology (PNI) looks at the connection between our minds, hormonal systems, and the functioning of the immune system and tissues of the body. It has shown, without any shadow of doubt, that stress definitely alters the activity not only of the immune system but also of all other tissues. What has been found is that there are receptors on all the cells of the body for brain messenger chemicals called neuropeptides which, when activated, can either excite or depress cell functioning.

In those who are stressed and depressed, immune and other tissue functioning can be markedly depressed too, influencing both the number of circulating immune cells and their individual activity. This can put people at risk of infections and other illnesses, and it is very likely that prolonged stress or severe shock and upset can allow abnormal cancer cells (which would normally be spotted and destroyed) to escape surveillance and survive. However, the degree of cellular and immune system depression does vary greatly between individuals who are experiencing similar levels of stress. It now appears clear from other psychological and PNI studies that the key determinant is not how much stress or upset we have but how we respond to it.

It has been shown that the immune system is able to learn responses or become programmed to key triggers. Thus it is likely that those who were sensitized in early life to loss, grief, powerlessness and anxiety and have suppressed their emotional response to these problems, have a particularly pronounced psychological and immunological reaction to subsequent problems. Some people will therefore be more at risk due to their psychological make-up and history. This may well be the reason why population studies do not show clear-cut results in relation to stress and adverse life events and cancer incidence. However, it is very likely that the general increase in stress in society from high-pressure living is weakening our immune systems, which could be a significant factor in the increasing incidence of cancer. This picture of individualized stress-risk factors parallels within a bigger picture the situation with chemicals and cancer – there are chemicals which affect us all but which are particularly risky to those with a specific vulnerability to them.

In time, no doubt the true extent of the risks created by psychological factors will be known and the potential role of the mind in helping us to survive and prevent cancer will be understood. It will not be long before we are able to screen and monitor individuals for the effects of stress on their body tissue and immune function. Using this information, we will be able to offer protective psychological strategies to those who are especially vulnerable. In the meantime, because of this new scientific work and the experience of the Bristol Cancer Help Centre and other cancer support centres, we currently have enough understanding of the huge importance of psychological health and mind–body techniques in cancer to include the mind–body element fairly and squarely in advice on cancer prevention.

WHICH ARE THE MOST COMMON CANCERS?

Statistics from the Cancer Registry, 1997			
In men:			
Type of Cancer	*% by age 65*	*Over lifetime*	*Lifetime risk*
Lung	1.7	8.0	1 in 13
Prostate	0.9	7.3	1 in 14
Colorectal	1.4	5.7	1 in 18
Bladder	0.7	3.3	1 in 30
Stomach	0.5	2.3	1 in 44
Oesophageal	0.4	1.3	1 in 75
Kidney	0.4	1.1	1 in 89
Leukaemia	0.4	1.1	1 in 94
Pancreatic	0.3	1.0	1 in 96

In women:			
Type of Cancer	% by age 65	Over lifetime	Lifetime risk
Breast	5.6	10.9	1 in 9
Colorectal	1.1	4.9	1 in 20
Lung	0.4	4.3	1 in 23
Ovarian	0.9	2.1	1 in 48
Uterine	0.6	1.4	1 in 73
Bladder	0.2	1.3	1 in 79
Stomach	0.2	1.2	1 in 86
Pancreatic	0.2	1.1	1 in 95
Cervical	0.6	0.9	1 in 116

It is very clear from these statistics how much the risk of cancer increases over the age of 65. With life expectancy increasing all the time, we must all take steps now to prevent ourselves suffering from cancer when we are older, so that our potentially 'golden years' do not become a misery.

RISK FACTORS FOR SPECIFIC CANCERS

There is considerable variation in the risk factors for different cancers. A list of the risk factors for the most common cancers can be found in Appendix 2.

Who is at risk?

With the emphasis that has been put over the past decade on the importance of genetic factors in the development of cancer, the public could not be blamed for thinking that the disease is largely an inherited one. But, in fact, as we have already heard, a family history of cancer only accounts for between 1 and 5 per cent of all cancers. Even in this small group of genetic cancers, we need to ask ourselves if lifestyle and environmental pollution play a part in activating cancer genes. In reality, these cancer genes have always existed and it is highly likely that poor diet and toxic lifestyles are now causing these oncogenes to express themselves increasingly frequently. Don't forget, cancer-prone genes still need to undergo at least one or two mutations before they become activated oncogenes or 'cancer genes'. It is therefore very important that we do not fall back into a sense of impotence, thinking that cancer is an inherited disease about which we can do very little.

At the year 2001, eleven cancer-prone genes have been discovered which are involved in normal cell growth and division which can, if mutated, lead to the development of: chronic myeloid leukaemia; lymphoid neoplasms; chronic lymphatic leukaemia; Birkett's lymphoma; cancer of the breast, ovaries, bladder, stomach, lung, cervix, colon, pancreas, genito-urinary tract, colon and thyroid; squamous head and neck tumours; melanomas (skin cancer); and endocrine (or glandular) cancers.

There are a further seventeen tumour-suppresser genes which, if mutated, can become involved in the development of: cancers of the colon, duodenum (small intestine), lymph, breast, ovaries, prostate, pancreas, uterus, urinary tract, kidney, brain and thyroid; pheochromacytoma (cancer of the adrenal gland), sarcomas (cancers of the bones or connective tissues), melanomas, leukaemias, retinoblastoma (tumour of the retina in the back of the eye), osteosarcoma and haemangioblastoma (cancer of the blood vessel walls). Despite this huge list of cancers in which these oncogenes can be implicated, it is important to remember that most cancers arise from the longer five- or six-step process which occurs in previously normal tissue (described in the section on how cancer develops page 17)

From this overview of the causes of cancer, it is clear that a combination of occupation and lifestyle can have a very big influence on your likelihood of getting the disease. Overall, the factor which increases the incidence of cancer the most is age. The longer we live, our chance of developing cancer increases dramatically. This is due to a combination of many of the factors mentioned earlier – an accumulation of toxins in the body over time leading to an increase in genetic mutation, decreasing physical activity, obesity, hormone replacement therapy, medical procedures, smoking, alcohol and, in general, a decrease in the reliability of cellular function and regulatory mechanisms, especially when nutrition has been poor with a processed and overrich Western diet.

Because modern medicine and health improvements enable people to live longer we now have a society with a large number of elderly people. As the population ages, there is an associated rise in cancer incidence and, therefore, mortality. However, there are also worrying increases in cancer incidence among younger people, especially smoking-related cancers in women and childhood leukaemias.

The other major factors which affect cancer incidence are nationality, culture and social and societal trends. In fact, it has been the study of this disease in different populations which has shed so much light on the causes of cancer and the possibility of preventing it. It is not easy to persuade people to change or to get societies to adopt wholesale the values and customs of others. However, gaining insight from the differing patterns of cancer incidence around the world can give us a vital starting place to understand the most important factors.

A good example of national variations can be seen in Japanese people, living in Japan, who have high stomach cancer rates but very low rates of breast cancer compared with people in the West. In the UK, a woman has around a one in nine lifetime chance of developing breast cancer, whereas in Japan it is closer to one in forty-five. This has been put down to the far lower incidence of obesity in Japanese women; the lower circulating levels of post-menopausal oestrogen; the extremely low intake of dairy foods and relatively low intake of meat, along with a high intake of soya products (which contain phyto-oestrogens) and the drinking of green tea. The phyto-oestrogens are very weak oestrogenic compounds which sit on and block the oestrogen hormone receptors, acting a bit like tamoxifen, the oestrogen-blocking drug. This is thought to protect Japanese women from the effects of circulating oestrogen, thus conveying significant protection against breast cancer. On the other hand, the Japanese diet includes large amounts of protein (particularly in the form of raw fish) as well as vegetable pickles and salted foods. These predispose the Japanese to a high level of stomach cancer.

Sadly, however, once Japanese women forsake their traditional culture for a Western lifestyle, their protection against breast cancer is lost. Japanese people who move to the United States, for example, develop the lower stomach cancer and higher breast cancer rates of US Caucasians within only five years of arriving.

In some developing countries, cancer is much more likely to be caused by infectious agents, and it is already known that liver cancer is associated with the intake of aflatoxin. It is also clear that in Africa, where rural communities eat mainly high-fibre vegetarian diets, there are very low levels of both hormonal and gastric cancers. On the other hand, sexually transmitted cancers such as cervical cancer are far more common.

The gravest concern for the developing world is that posed by the wholesale adoption of Western lifestyles. People within traditional cultures need to be informed as a matter of urgency about the severe health risks associated with a Western lifestyle and diet and given strong reinforcement of the healthy aspects of their traditional lifestyles. There is a great risk that the media image of Western success will overtake and smother traditional values, wiping out many unique cultures and placing many people's health at great risk.

For the Western world, the challenge is to prevent a significant rise in viral cancers of the cervix, liver and blood, caused by a combination of poor nutrition, poverty, drug addiction (through the use of non-sterile needles) and unsafe sex.

CONVENTIONAL CANCER TREATMENT

Despite the billions of pounds and dollars that have been poured into cancer research oyer the past fifty years and the enormous increase in our understanding of the way cancer develops, medical treatment still remains woefully ineffective in offering hope of a cure to the majority of people with the disease. Realistically, the possibility of a cure can be offered only to those with three of the relatively rarer cancers – testicular cancer and some of the lymphomas and leukaemias.

Cancer medicine does not greatly alter the long-term prognosis in any of the common cancers (of the lung, breast, bowel and prostate), where the major role of conventional treatment is to delay spread of the disease and increase what is known as the 'disease-free interval'. This means symptoms and signs of the illness are temporarily removed so that the person with cancer can enjoy a relatively normal life for longer, until the return of the disease eventually makes death inevitable. Newer medical approaches are beginning to offer some promising increases in life expectancy but, compared to the amount of work that has gone into trying to achieve these ends, the results are disappointing. The conventional treatments for cancer are typically:

- surgery, to remove the tumour (where it is a solid tumour rather than a blood cancer).

- radiotherapy, where radiation is used after surgery to

destroy stray cells around the operation site that may have been missed during surgery, or to treat inoperable cancers or cancer secondaries which may be causing severe local problems such as nerve or arterial compression.

- chemotherapy, which involves giving drugs that destroy rapidly dividing cells (rapid division is the main feature distinguishing cancer cells from other cells in the body, although other rapidly dividing tissue such as skin, nails, hair, the gut lining and immune and other blood cells may also be damaged in the process)

- adjuvant hormone blocking therapy, given in cancers of the breast and prostate to block female and male hormones which stimulate the tumour's growth.

It is the relative lack of efficacy of cancer medicine and the very rigorous nature of these treatments (which in themselves can produce second cancers) that make the issue of prevention so absolutely vital. For this reason, and because cancer is such a serious and unpleasant disease, it is imperative that the prevention and eradication of cancer moves to the very top of our personal, professional and societal agendas.

THE STATE OF CANCER RESEARCH

The majority of the cancer research budget in the UK, mainland Europe and the United States is currently dedicated to investigating how cancer develops and to the treatment of cancer. A very small proportion of the budget is spent on researching prevention or, more importantly, on the implementation of cancer prevention strategies. We already have enough key information to eradicate a large proportion of preventable cancer. Certainly, the American National Breast Cancer Coalition has discovered that women with breast cancer feel that the very highest priority for cancer research should be prevention, not treatment.

At present by far the biggest proportion of cancer research budgets worldwide goes into research on the role of genetics in cancer formation. The hope is that by understanding properly how cancer develops, doctors will be able to formulate better treatment strategies. Currently, on the treatment side, a lot of work is focused on developing mechanisms to target chemotherapy drugs that will work only on the cancer itself and not affect other tissues. There is also work under way to see if genetically modified viruses can be used to correct genetic abnor malities in cancer cells, as well as other techniques to repair defective DNA. Many other trials are comparing the efficacy of different mixtures and types of chemotherapy drugs.

The other big push currently among UK cancer research charities is for studies in the use of the hormone-blocking drug tamoxifen to prevent breast cancer in healthy women. As mentioned previously, this avenue of research has its opponents.

Almost weekly we see press reports of important cancer breakthroughs but, in reality, these usually amount to tiny clues in a massive jigsaw. They are often laboratory findings in animal studies which may or may not be found to relate to human cancer development or treatment.

Encouragingly, in the UK, a large-scale trial – the European Prospective Investigation into Cancer and Nutrition – is looking in depth at the relationship between diet and cancer. In the UK alone, 25,000 men and women have been recruited for this study, and their dietary patterns and cancer incidence will be compared with that of a further 400,000 people in mainland Europe in order to assess the incidence of cancer in relation to different eating patterns. Another study is looking at whether a daily intake of the mineral selenium can reduce cancer incidence – this link is being investigated because there are more cancer cases in areas where the soil is lower in selenium and early findings are promising.

In the United States, the potential role of alternative and complementary therapies is also being taken seriously at last. The American National Institute of Health has set up an office of Alternative Medicines, which in turn is currently setting up research centres for all areas of medicine. The centre for the study of alternative and complementary medicine in cancer is located at the University of Houston, Texas. There, they are studying the effectiveness of different herbs, vitamins, mineral supplements and foods when used with orthodox treatment, as well as studying them in their own right for cancer treatment and palliative care.

The reality of the situation, as stated in 1998 by Professor Karol Sikora, formerly of the World Health Organization's Department of Cancer Strategy, is that it is unlikely that the treatment of cancer will ever be the solution to the problem. We must therefore wake up and focus all our efforts on cancer prevention and heed the message that the rising incidence of cancer is giving us about our societal and environmental problems. We must look forward with hope to the great personal and social rewards of tackling cancer at source. We must not passively accept cancer as part of life whilst we watch the effects of this dreadful Western disease spread inexorably through our friends and family, and into developing countries where there are no resources whatsoever to deal with the problem.

Professor Sikora's message brings home how important it is to exert our personal and professional will in tackling this disease; simultaneously we must confront personal and global apathy as we witness that which is most precious to us becoming corrupted and fatally threatened. It is important to recognize that the PR messages of the cancer charities, telling us of the great breakthroughs being made daily, are vital to their own survival and on-going work (important and laudable as that may be), but might be keeping us focused on the wrong priorities – those of cause and treatment rather than prevention. We must not hope just to treat cancer, we must hope to eradicate it, and the way to do that is through cancer prevention.

CANCER POLITICS

If you were the Prime Minister today, faced with the reality that cancer is a problem created by cigarettes,

Western diet, alcohol, the chemical industry, intensive farming and environmental pollution, not to mention the medical profession, you might feel ever so slightly daunted by the prospect of trying to eradicate it! To take on the combined might of the tobacco, alcohol, pharmaceutical, petrochemical and agricultural industries, plus the medical profession, would be immediate suicide for any politician.

During the heat of the initial BSE crisis in the mid-1990s, the Committee on the Medical Aspects of Food was also sitting, reviewing evidence about the relationship between cancer and diet. The findings of doctors Key and Thorogood – that vegetarians were 40 to 50 per cent less likely to die of cancer than meat eaters – had been published in 1994, but it took this committee until 1998 to make the public recommendation that meat eating was definitely associated with increased cancer risk. Not surprisingly, the release of the committee's findings was not made public until the heat had gone out of the first wave of the BSE crisis.

In 1996, when asked face to face why the British Government was not taking a more direct approach to this link between cancer and diet, the then Secretary of State for Health replied quite unashamedly: 'How could we – the farmers would kill us!'.

It is extremely difficult for any government with a short term of office and its eye on the next election to make the kind of decisions that will truly protect the health of the nation. Successive governments focus on achieving health targets through the improvement of medicine rather than tackling the core root of the problem of degenerative illness. It is likely that whilst medicine is firmly in the grip of the pharmaceutical companies and governments are firmly in the hands of industry and market forces, we will never see policies being made which address the problem of cancer head-on. Instead, present-day governments are focusing on healthy-living initiatives within the community that will put the responsibility for leading healthy lives back into our own hands.

This means that it is up to all of us as individuals to take charge ourselves – in our family group, in our places of work, in our institutions and local communities – and to put in place, step by step, the behavioural changes, policies and practices which will systematically eradicate cancer from our lives and from our society. As more and more healthy-living initiatives develop, giving support particularly to the most disadvantaged in society, the great hope is that the public will be empowered and enabled to make healthy choices, and that the incidence of cancer will drop steadily over the years to come.

CHAPTER 2: CLEANING UP YOUR ACT

ELIMINATING POTENTIAL CAUSES OF CANCER

This chapter contains specific advice on how to eliminate potential causes of cancer from your life. Considerable emphasis is given to getting the necessary support and help to change the habits of a lifetime, especially when these habits represent emotional crutches 'to get you through the day' such as unhealthy use of food, alcohol and cigarettes.

The main issues to address in relation to food and cancer are:

- obesity

- foods and food additives

- cooking methods

Obesity

Obesity has already been linked to an increased risk of cancer of the breast, endometrium (womb lining), gall bladder and large bowel, and is likely to be linked to cancer of the prostate, ovaries, kidney and pancreas.

Obesity is measured by calculating Body Mass Index (BMI) – see page 33. The World Health Organization (WHO) defines obesity as a BMI greater than 30, overweight as a BMI of 25 or over, and desirable weight as a BMI of between 20 and 25.

World Health Organization Weight Categories			
BMI:	20–24.9	25–29.9	30–40	greater than 40
Description:	desirable weight	overweight	obese	severely obese

Obesity levels in developed countries are rising at alarming rates. While the US has the worst obesity record, the UK is rapidly catching up (see below).

Percentage of overweight and obese people in England in 1998			
	% Overweight	% Obese	Total
Men	45.5	17.3	62.8
Women	32.1	21.2	53.3
Percentage of overweight and obese children (at age 6 and 15) in the UK in 1996			
	% Overweight	% Obese	Total
Boys aged 6	22.1	11.7	33.8
Boys aged 15	32.9	16.4	49.3
Girls aged 6	21.5	9	30.5
Girls aged 15	28.8	17.3	46.1

The obesity problem in the UK has increased dramatically over the last two decades. While in 1980, 8 per cent of women and 6 per cent of men were obese, today rates have risen to 21.2 per cent and 17.3 per cent respectively. This means that in only twenty years the prevalence of obesity has tripled. However, the UK still falls behind the US, where over a third of the adult population are obese, rising to more than 50 per cent in some ethnic subgroups. What is apparent, though, is that rates of increase in obesity levels have been similar in the US and the UK over the last two decades. This offers a frightening insight into the potential scale of the problem in the UK unless adequate preventative strategies are adopted now.

Obesity is a risk factor not only for cancer. People who are overweight are at higher risk of all the degenerative diseases – especially those of the cardiovascular system and joints. Hopefully, by understanding that obesity is a serious risk factor for cancer as well as heart disease, you will finally feel compelled to do something about your own weight (if necessary), diet and the diet of those around you.

If current trends continue, it is estimated that by 2005, 20 per cent of men and 23 per cent of women in the UK will be obese. In developing countries, affluence is associated with obesity, and obesity can, indeed, be considered desirable. However, in developed countries, the opposite is true. Obesity rates are much higher in lower social classes than in professional groups. In the UK, serious obesity levels go up from 10.7 per cent among the well-off in social class 1 to 25.3 per cent among those living in poverty.

On a global level, the International Obesity Task Force (IOTF), under the auspices of the WHO, has been formed to tackle the issue (see Appendix 1). Its aims are to:

- raise awareness at all levels that obesity is a serious medical condition and a major global health problem.

- develop policy recommendations for a coherent and effective global approach to manage and prevent obesity.

- identify and implement strategies in collaboration with experts, professional organizations, patient groups and national health agencies.

Tackling the problem of excess weight

Finding out if you are overweight or obese is the first step to tackling the problem. You may like to calculate your BMI (see page 33) and work out which of the WHO categories you come into (see the table above). This will give you a clear indication of how urgent the problem is for you personally.

If your BMI falls into the obese or severely obese categories, it may well be possible to receive help and support in losing weight from your GP or a specialist. However, in the UK, there are currently only six obesity clinics offering specialist help and so people with weight problems often find themselves on their own. If this is the case, you can seek help from the voluntary sector. Getting the right sort of help will be discussed below in the section 'How we eat'.

Even if you are overweight rather than obese, I would

urge you strongly to act now to take your weight and diet in hand. Whilst it is extremely important not to let self-esteem suffer as a result of being overweight, it is vital for health, well-being and quality of life that this issue is tackled head-on. As well as considering your own weight, it is also important to extend your concern about healthy eating and the avoidance of obesity to places of work, schools, hospitals, prisons and care homes. If you are involved in the management of any of these organizations, or are a user of any of these facilities, get involved in making sure that the organization urgently adopts a healthy eating policy. A good place to start is by replacing easy access to sweets, crisps and sugary drinks with access to fruit, fruit juices, wholefood snacks and mineral water.

The causes of obesity

There are a few very rare situations in which the causes of obesity are medical. But for the vast majority obesity comes down to:

- the foods we eat

- how much we eat

- how we eat

The foods we eat

Fat, sugar and alcohol

Fat, refined sugars and alcohol are the biggest offenders in the onset of obesity. Most people in developed countries effectively double their calorie intake each day by eating sweets, sugary drinks and fatty snacks such as crisps, and by drinking alcohol. All these items are superfluous to our body's requirements, making us fat and lethargic and putting our health at risk. Another problem is that these are empty calories which take away our hunger and reduce our appetite for proper healthy foods which contain the vital vitamins, minerals and plant phytochemicals required for protection against cancer. A further problem is that a sudden rise in blood-sugar, fat or alcohol levels in the bloodstream puts the body into physiological stress, and all (particularly brain) tissue function is potentially lethally threatened. The body's rebalancing mechanisms then have to work very hard to restore equilibrium, a process which uses up a lot of precious vitamins and minerals.

So by snacking on these foods, people can end up both obese and depleted in vital nutrients. Growing children, the sick and the elderly are at greatest risk because they can often be tempted with sweet foods and fizzy drinks which have virtually no nutritional value whatsoever, only 'empty calories'. These nutrition-poor foods will particularly affect growth, brain development, ageing and resistance to disease.

Fried foods

The next biggest offender is fried food, eaten both in the home and in fast-food outlets. It is virtually impossible to buy healthy food in these places, where the main emphasis is on burgers, fish and chips, and children's snacks covered in batter and breadcrumbs such as 'chicken nuggets'. To make things worse, most children's meals from fast-food outlets have no vegetables with them at all other than chips. As mentioned earlier it has been estimated that 47 per cent of inner-city children eat no vegetables other than chips.

Often adults who cook vegetables and make salads for themselves will happily feed their children on a regular diet of burgers, fish fingers and pizzas with chips. This is often followed by ice cream, and is washed down with fizzy, sweetened drinks. We then wonder why so many children become sickly, irritable and obese and under-achieve at school!

Animal fats and meat

The emphasis on meat and animal fats in the Western diet plays a major role in obesity. Heavy use of cheese, meat, butter, cream and yoghurt has disastrous consequences on our health and weight. In Oriental cultures, where there is a far higher use of rice, grains and vegetables, with protein and animal fat being used in smaller quantities, obesity levels are practically non-existent.

How much we eat

Working out how much we eat – both at meal times and in snacks during the day – is an important start to tackling obesity. Keeping a food diary for a week is one way of monitoring eating patterns. When it is written down in black and white, the amount you actually eat can be quite shocking. Because access to snacks at home, at work and on the high street is so easy for most people these days – not to mention the almost 24-hour-availability of sweets and chocolates in garages, supermarkets, theatres and cinemas – it is easy to be munching all the time. Guidelines state that children should have around 1750 calories a day, women around 2000 and men around 2500 if they have a fairly sedentary lifestyle, which is the norm in this day and age. The total calories required will vary according to the height and occupation of the person. On an affluent Western diet it is very easy to consume in excess of the entire daily calorie allowance in one meal. For example, with pre-meal drinks and peanuts, an hors-d'oeuvre such as pâté with bread and butter, a main meal such as steak and chips, a cheesecake pudding, coffee, chocolates, not to mention two glasses of wine and two pints of beer, you would consume 3750 calories! Or a child who consumes two bags of crisps, three cans of fizzy drink and a chocolate bar will have consumed 1000 calories without any proper food at all.

It also seems to be true that the more we eat the more we want to eat. We get used to eating large meals on a regular basis, and if portions get larger then the amount we need in order to feel satisfied gets greater, and the vicious circle continues. Because people are aware they may eat excessively during the evenings or when they go out, another problem creeps in – the diet/binge phe-nomenon. People often starve themselves all day so that they can go out and eat a huge meal in the evening. There is a lot of evidence to suggest that this type of famine-and-feast routine is counterproductive in terms of putting on weight. In response to the famine phase our bodies go into a very low and efficient basal metabolic rate, hanging on to our weight and burning off calories very slowly. Then as the calories come rushing in during the feast, the body goes straight into fat-storage mode in case there is more famine on the way! It is therefore definitely not a good idea to adopt this type of strategy for weight control. There is also evidence that if we eat the majority of our calories at the end of the day when there is no chance to exercise, more fat is deposited throughout the night than would be if the equivalent amount of food was eaten at breakfast or lunchtime.

When we snack or 'graze' continuously, we hardly ever feel hungry. When we eat very large meals we become used to overriding the initial feelings of fullness and satisfaction and go on eating way beyond what we actually need. To become healthy it is terribly important that we start again, tuning into ourselves and learning what our bodies really need, rather than eating too much out of habit.

So, to avoid obesity we must:

- reduce the amount of calories in each meal, keeping within the daily calorie allowance.

- avoid snacks between meals other than fruit and whole-food cereal biscuits.

- eat regular meals, spreading calorie intake evenly throughout the day.

- avoid eating the bulk of calories at the end of the day.

How we eat
For many people in the West, consumption of food has come to have very little to do with hunger. Much of what

we eat is either for pure sensory gratification (to provide us with emotional comfort or sedation or to cover our nervousness) or in social contexts. Rich, fatty foods dampen anxiety and emotional stress because blood flow to the digestive system is temporarily prioritized away from the brain and muscles. This is why we feel sleepy after a big meal and are advised not to swim soon after eating. There is nothing wrong with food being a great source of sensory delight, but it is vital we learn how to cook and choose foods which are good for us and low in calories. This kind of food can be made equally delightful once we acquire the necessary knowledge and develop the right skills. Detailed attention will be given in Chapter 3 on how to go about converting our way of eating to a healthy one without losing any of the appeal and satisfaction.

The emotional and social reasons for what we eat are far more difficult to confront. Many people are aware they 'comfort eat' when they are lonely, depressed or anxious. Others comfort eat without realizing what they are doing. Family or institutional regimes with set meal times and set menus of many courses can make people adopt a way of eating that does not necessarily suit their constitution or appetite. In a family situation, pushy relatives may continually try to 'feed up' their partners or dependants, deriving satisfaction (and an element of control) from this care-giving role. In the meantime their loved ones become overweight, sedated and addicted to the wrong foods.

Another factor is that eating and drinking has become a major recreational activity in the West. As recently as the 1960s, in the UK a meal out was a special occasion. But today eating out is a weekly if not daily event for many people. This creates a different kind of emotional dependence on food – namely, feeling that you haven't had a good time unless socializing has involved the consumption of food.

During the 1980s we were briefly exposed to the influence of Nouvelle Cuisine and Cuisine Minceur, which emphasized quality over quantity, as well as delicacy and beauty in the presentation of food. However, this style of cooking concentrated on giving smaller portions of the same types of food, such as fish and meat with tiny amounts of vegetables and starch. As a result, many people were left feeling dissatisfied and hungry after handing over large quantities of cash! Understandably, people returned pretty quickly to the normal kinds of restaurant meals they had been used to before.

Changing our emotional and social eating patterns takes enormous focus and determination and a great deal of support. That is why most attempts to change our health simply through health promotion fail. Many people have the information about what is good or bad for them but do not have sufficient motivation or support to make the necessary changes.

The emotional element

To find out if there is a large emotional element to your way of eating, consider whether you:

- eat more when you are anxious, depressed or lonely.

- feel really bad if you cannot get access to food.

- reward yourself with food when you have done something difficult.

- get very anxious if food is late or there is a possibility someone else will eat the food allocated to you.

- binge on certain foods at times or have rituals and routines around shopping and food.

In simple terms, the use of food for comfort eating is linked to a need for emotional contact, love, support, touch, communication and security. The way to change a dependency on food is to find ways of meeting these needs directly, rather than indirectly with food.

Sometimes the link between emotions and foods goes beyond purely comfort eating and moves into the realm of an 'eating disorder'. This can result in someone becoming either overweight or, more commonly, underweight. If this is the case with you and you feel your eating habits are out of control, ruling your life or endangering you in some way, it may well be time to seek psychological or psychiatric help, as well as help to bring your weight under control. Either way, if you can recognize how you are using food and reach out for the help and support you need rather than food, the problem can eventually be sorted out.

It may be possible to try to do this yourself if you have good friends, family or a helpful partner around who are willing and able to give you the support and love you need. However, if you are isolated, it may be that you will need the help of a professional counsellor or support group to try to deal with these emotional needs in a different and more healthy way. There are a great number of support groups to help people lose weight, the most well known of which is Weight Watchers (see Appendix 1). Some groups focus mainly on dietary regimes with goals and rewards for losing weight, whilst others are more psychologically orientated, attempting to fill the gap left by letting go of excessive food consumption. Others focus on the use of a product to help with appetite suppression so that you don't need to eat so much. However, if the underlying emotional needs are not addressed, these techniques will only be a temporary solution. This means that getting help from a counsellor and joining the right kind of support group is usually the only way to make real long-term changes.

The other way of helping yourself emotionally is to come at the problem from the other direction and work on your emotional state through the use of self-help techniques such as relaxation, meditation, yoga and tai chi. These techniques will help to calm the mind and emotions and enable you to develop inner strength. Once your mind is calmer and stronger and more peaceful, you will have far more control and choice over how you behave. Developing any sort of exercise routine will help psychologically as well as physically, lifting the emotional state whilst throwing off unwanted calories. Again, this is OK if you have the discipline and support to exercise by yourself, but if this is hard for you to achieve find yourself a partner or 'buddy' to do it with you. Of course, a healthy active sex life will also help, both physically and mentally!

The social element

Changing the social aspect of how we eat also requires strong commitment. This may well involve confronting a partner or parent who continually overfeeds you, or, indeed, taking a good look at yourself and the way you feed others. If the people who feed you will not change their way of cooking, then you need to exert great self-discipline and eat only appropriate amounts of suitable foods. This can be hurtful and difficult for both the provider and for you, but it may be the only way to show you are serious. Hopefully, longer term, taking a stand will prompt them to change their behaviour too.

When holding a party, it is even harder to change your eating patterns without thinking you are depriving your guests or being a poor host or hostess. This really requires a great deal of imagination, and perhaps even frank discussion with friends about what you are trying to do. A good start is to plan social events around another activity rather than eating. For example, you can meet friends to enjoy music, poetry, sport, games, a film or play, or even to meditate together. Of course, you can still provide some sort of food, but if it is the secondary rather than the primary focus, then food consumption will be far lower. This may well be a tougher call for women than for men, as many women define themselves very strongly by their role of cook and hostess and will need to find new ways to express their creativity and generosity.

So, to correct both the emotional and social element of how you eat, try to:

- ascertain if you are eating to fulfil emotional needs and if so find ways of meeting these needs more appropriately.

- take the emphasis away from food in social situations and place it instead on other activities.

Foods and food additives which increase cancer risk

The main foods to cut out of your diet to prevent cancer are:

- red meat (pork, beef, lamb)

- animal fats

- foods which are pickled, preserved, smoked or salted

- food additives

Red meat
The Western diet has become very protein-rich, with meals at home and in restaurants often focused on huge pieces of meat or fish with few vegetables other than for decoration. There has been a dramatic rise in meat consumption since the Second World War and with it has come a huge increase in degenerative diseases, affecting our circulatory systems, joints and muscles and contributing significantly to the problem of cancer.

It is not yet clear exactly how eating red meat is linked

to cancer. But it is certainly possible for amino acids in meat to be turned into carcinogenic nitrosamines by acids in the gut. If transit time in the gut is slow due to a low-fibre diet, these substances can cause damage to the cells in the bowel wall and to other tissues once they have been absorbed into the blood. However, this mechanism is responsible for only a proportion of bowel cancers. Ultimately, the link between cancer and red meat may be explained by viruses that are passed down the food chain. This could mean that the BSE crisis is just the tip of the iceberg. It is certainly extremely striking that the 1998 findings of the prospective study by doctors Key and Thorogood showed that vegetarians are 40 to 50 per cent less likely to die of cancer than meat eaters. This is a huge effect and it is urgent that we discover the underlying mechanism behind this link. Meanwhile, it is vital to cut down consumption of red meat to a minimum or eliminate it altogether.

The advice from the Government's Committee on the Medical Aspects of Food is to cut down meat consumption in your diet to no more than 100 grams (around 3 ounces) a day. This includes the meat in products such as sausage rolls and pies as well as meat itself. It is far better though, to avoid having meat every day, and if possible to eliminate it altogether from the diet. If you are especially fond of meat and unable to give it up completely, have a meat meal once a week, buying the best quality organic meat if possible. By doing this you will be putting quality before quantity and will really enjoy the occasional treat, knowing that overall you are protecting yourself and your family by making this key dietary change.

The other important factor is to be sure that whenever you do eat meat, you have it with vegetables or salad. The carcinogenic effects of meat are lessened by the presence of vitamins and other plant chemicals in vegetables within the gut and their fibre content ensures a rapid gut transit time for the meat, which is also protective.

Try not to do a straight swap by replacing red meat with chicken or fish. Whilst these are preferable forms of protein, there may still be a risk with excess consumption. Even more important, try not to replace meat with cheese. All cheese is very high in animal fat and a diet of pizza or pasta covered in cheese sauce will make matters worse, not better. The best move for those who feel inspired to 'go the whole way' is to become completely vegan and eliminate animal products from the diet altogether. The major protein sources then become beans, lentils, nuts and seeds, which give the ideal balance of protein and healthy fats. Almost everyone who does this says the improvement in their health, energy and well-being is quite remarkable, and they wish they had done it years ago!

Animal fats

Animal fats are major contributors to obesity but it also appears that they carry a risk of cancer in their own right. Therefore, as just mentioned, it is very important not to swap meat for cheese and other high-fat dairy products. The advice is to keep their consumption to a bare minimum. This means dramatically reducing consumption of cheese, butter, milk and cream and cutting down on yoghurt and eggs. It also means cutting the fat from meat, giving up cooking with any animal fats such as lard and suet, and keeping the use of butter or cream in cooking to a minimum. Animal fats for cooking should be replaced with vegetable oils, and enriching recipes with butter and cream should be avoided for this sort of cookery is at the root of the Western dietary and obesity problem.

There are certain fats which are vital to our health, called essential fatty acids. The most helpful of these are omega-3 fatty acids which are found in fish oils and linseed oil, as well as in many nuts and seeds. Linseed oil tablets can be taken or linseeds can be crushed and sprinkled over food to ensure an adequate intake of these vital fatty acids. Even with the healthier vegetable oils like olive oil, it is very important to avoid overconsumption of fat by their excessive use in dressings and cooking. This, too, will lead to obesity and all the associated health problems.

Foods including preservatives and additives

It is best to avoid all foods which have been pickled, smoked, salted or preserved with additives such as sodium nitrate (saltpetre) and others. Saltpetre can promote the formation of carcinogenic nitrosamines with the protein in preserved foods such as sausages and salami. Smoking food can also lead to the formation of carcinogenic, polycyclic aromatic hydrocarbons. Sadly, this means that both bacon and sausages, the staple ingredients of the traditional English breakfast, must go – or certainly become a very rare treat. On top of the additives in sausages and the harmful substances in smoked bacon, the high animal fat content of these foods and the superheating of these fats during cooking make them key items to avoid. We must all get ourselves converted to delicious healthy breakfasts of fresh fruit salads, cereals, porridge, pancakes and toast and give up our addiction to the big 'fry-up'.

The salting and pickling of food has been shown to produce higher levels of oesophageal and stomach cancer in Japan and of nose and throat cancer in China, and in both these countries there is a serious need to give up certain traditional dietary habits in favour of healthy new ones.

In general, food additives should be avoided, as should artificial sweeteners, which have also been linked to cancer. Although food additives have been shown to cause less than 1 per cent of cancers (along with other forms of environmental pollutants), nonetheless this should be enough to encourage us to eat wholefoods which do not contain additives. The advice here is to eat only fresh food, avoiding anything that is stored long term in jars or cans or that is 'enhanced' or preserved in any artificial way.

There is no need for people to eat preserved foods – such as bright-green, tinned mushy peas – in this day and age when fresh and frozen food is available in all seasons. Methods of preserving food artificially or heightening its appeal with false colours or flavours are unnecessary, and these foods should be eliminated from the diet and replaced with (preferably organic) wholefood, which is additive and preservative free.

Cooking methods which increase cancer risk

Cooking methods which should be avoided to reduce the risk of cancer are:

- char-grilling and barbecuing

- frying, especially in super-heated oils

- smoking

- microwaving (potentially)

Char-grilling and barbecuing

As delicious as they may be, char-grilled or barbecued meats are definitely associated with increased cancer risk. The parts of meat which become charred contain dangerous polycyclic aromatic hydrocarbons which can cause DNA damage. Unfortunately, this means we should throw out our barbecues and restrain ourselves from ordering char-grilled foods in restaurants! Home barbecuing has shot up in popularity over the last ten years and barbecues are now available in every hardware store and garden centre and charcoal is sold at most large garages and supermarkets. Barbecues have become associated with good times and a party atmosphere, and barbecued food is becoming increasingly available in pub and restaurant gardens and at outdoor events. Sadly, this is a trend we must reverse in order to help prevent cancer.

Advice in other literature suggests that if people are going to eat barbecued or char-grilled food, they should first take some vitamin C, betacarotene and other anti-oxidant vitamins and minerals to protect themselves. This seems a good idea but it is much better to avoid these foods in the first place. Again, as with the advice for red meat, if you do eat char-grilled or barbecued food, it is vital to have plenty of vegetables and salad with it – not just the customary lettuce leaf and half a tomato as garnish we so often see when eating out.

An added source of danger when barbecuing is the toxic starter fuel which is often poured all over the charcoal in order to get the fire started or to keep it going. If meat is placed on the barbecue before the fuel has been fully burnt off, the volatile fuel vapour evaporates quickly in the smoke and can be absorbed into its fat. When the meat is eaten, this chemical can then be absorbed into our system. It is therefore important when using these fuels to make sure they are completely burnt off before putting any food on the barbecue, being especially careful if more fuel is added later in the cooking process to get the charcoal going again.

Frying
Frying is to be avoided as much as possible because the high temperatures involved can break down the fats into carcinogenic free radicals. It is particularly important to avoid heating cooking oils and fats until they smoke and the use of animal fats such as lard or dripping should definitely be avoided because of the high level of saturated fats. Also avoid re-using old oil for deep-frying as this will degenerate every time it is used. In fact, it is much better to abandon deep-frying and deep fried foods

altogether as they are extremely fattening and therefore convey risk for cancer and heart disease. Safer ways of frying such as stir-frying and even water frying are described in the section on healthy cooking methods on page 204.

Smoking
As with char-grilling and barbecuing, the smoking of food can cause dangerous changes to the proteins or fats in fish and meat. It is therefore wise to cut out smoked foods in order to reduce the risk of cancer.

Microwaving
There is no direct evidence as yet linking microwaved foods to an increased cancer risk. However, as explained in Chapter 1, microwaving heats food to a very high level, causing unnecessary destruction of vital nutrients whilst leaving food dangerously hot. The excessive heat is likely to damage the lining of the mouth, oesophagus and stomach if proper standing times for microwaved foods are not observed. It is therefore not advisable to use a microwave – because of its effect on the nutritional value of foods and because it breaks down the vitamins, plant enzymes and phytochemicals which can protect against cancer. It is early days to know for sure whether the use of microwaves in itself is safe, but certainly it is vital that manufacturers' instructions are followed to the letter. Ideally, we should eliminate the microwave cooker from our lives and return to more traditional cooking methods.

Smoking

The message about smoking and cancer could not be clearer. Smoking of any sort should be stopped, whether it is cigarette, pipe or cigar smoking. It is also important not to chew tobacco or inhale tobacco products as snuff. As well as giving up smoking, it is extremely important to keep away from other people's smoke – at home, at work or when socializing. Make it absolutely clear to friends and family that your home and car are no-smoking areas. Campaign to make your place of work a smoke-free area if humanly possible. Sit in no-smoking areas of trains and public buildings and always ask specifically to be seated in the no-smoking area in restaurants. The more this is demanded, the greater the allocation of space for non-smokers will be. If you are in charge at work or at any place where the public meet, take a stand and declare it a no-smoking zone.

Most important, though, is the need to be responsible around children. Never smoke in front of children or pregnant women, or if you are pregnant yourself. It is completely wrong that the environment of a child, born or unborn, should be polluted in this way. Children should never be put at increased risk of lung disease and cancer by adults who smoke.

There is very encouraging news from Sir Richard Doll and Sir Richard Peto from the Imperial Cancer Research Fund's Oxford unit that widespread cessation of smoking in the UK has already halved the number of lung cancer deaths in 2000 (by comparison with Doll's 1950 results). The study found that of men who continue to smoke, 16 per cent will die before 75 but for those who stop before 50 the rate goes down to 6 per cent. For those who stop before 30 it is less than 2 per cent. In 1950 the UK had the worst lung cancer death rates in the world but has had the best decrease since then. Lung cancer death rates are also falling rapidly in the US although the drop came much later than in the UK. Since 1970 the American lung cancer death rate has also halved in middle aged men. However, this compares starkly to the overall world-wide picture because of the rise in lung cancer deaths in developing countries. There were 100 million tobacco deaths in the world in the twentieth century and if smoking continues to increase at today's rates it is predicted that there will be 1,000 million in the twenty-first century.

Giving up

In developed countries everyone knows that smoking is dangerous and yet many people continue to smoke. This is another example of how information alone does not change behaviour. To give up smoking, both nicotine addiction and emotional dependency on smoking have to be addressed. While nicotine is admittedly very addictive, most people who smoke are as 'hooked' emotionally as they are chemically.

Nicotine addiction

Usually, after stopping smoking the withdrawal effects from nicotine last only a few days and the chemical craving is likely to be gone within a week or two. If you feel you are chemically dependent on cigarettes it is possible to get help with nicotine patches, nicotine chewing gum or even nicotine inhalers. These give a sub-stitute nicotine 'fix' and mean you can wean yourself off nicotine slowly, knowing that you are protected mean-while from the carcinogens in tobacco smoke. However, doing it this way just puts off the 'evil hour' when you must break the link and give up the nicotine dependency.

Emotional dependency

Ultimately, success in giving up smoking will almost invariably revolve around being sufficiently motivated and having the right level of support emotionally. So, it is in these areas where we should really focus our efforts.

Most smokers smoke because it helps them to control difficult feelings of anxiety, nervousness, self-conscious-ness, upset, loneliness, anger or grief. Nicotine is a stim-ulant which gives people a slight lift. The physiological changes brought about by tobacco smoke temporarily change their state of mind, blotting out to some extent the feelings they had before they picked up a cigarette, pipe or cigar. The problem is that this is a very tempo-rary lift and, because of the other harmful effects of cig-arettes, it often leaves people feeling more irritable or anxious than before. As with all other drugs, the simple solution is then to have more, and so the vicious circle continues.

Because of the underlying emotional reasons why people smoke, it is ridiculous to think that either good advice or even scaring people with medical data will make a big difference to their habit. The increasing number of therapeutic and self-help services, both private and voluntary, in the community means more people now have the chance to understand their underlying state of mind. Working on improving our state of mind and emotions depends on:

- allowing ourselves to recognize, feel and express emotions.

- being able to make our needs known clearly and ask for what we need.

- feeling safe and secure through the development of loving relationships.

- developing a loving and nurturing relationship with ourselves.

- developing inner strength and calmness through self-help techniques such as relaxation, meditation, visualization, yoga and tai chi.

- developing outlets for creativity and self-expression.

Quite often, changing underlying psychological problems requires some 'emotional re-education'. If people need to suppress their emotions with cigarettes, they are likely to have grown up in environments where it was unsafe or seen as just plain embarrassing to express how they felt. Support and encouragement are required and sometimes permission needs to be given in order for feelings to be felt and expressed. It is hard to change emotional habits or patterns on your own and it may well take half a dozen sessions with a counsellor to experience a different way of dealing with your feelings. Counselling help is particularly good if you time it so that you have a couple of sessions before giving up and then continue during the crucial period when you are first coming off cigarettes, when emotions that have been suppressed long term through smoking may come up to the surface.

Another way of getting help is to join a support group, where you will be given the opportunity to talk about how you feel. Obviously, these groups offer less direct one-to-one support and so may not be enough for some people. Support agencies exist throughout the UK to help people who want to stop smoking (see Appendix 1).

In a good counselling relationship, people are able to let go and express their feelings, learn how to deal with emotions differently, develop a new nurturing relationship with themselves and develop a positive relationship with the counsellor on which they can model other good relationships in the future. They are also able to explore the whole question of expressing themselves fully and reaching their potential in life. In this situation, people learn how to communicate well and how to explore and define their needs, but sometimes they need to take the process further by seeking out assertiveness training. If you are too shy or embarrassed to voice your feelings and needs, often finding yourself bullied or overwhelmed and resorting to smoking to calm yourself, these classes would be a very good idea. You will be trained in techniques that will, first, help you to identify what it is you are feeling and needing, and, second, teach you to express your need clearly and repeatedly until it is met. As well as being able to control the frustration and hurt involved in continually being trampled on, you will find other knock-on benefits with these techniques.

Developing inner strength

This idea has already been mentioned in the section on emotional dependency on food. It is worth re-emphasizing the point that it is possible to make an enormous difference to your state of mind through yoga, yoga breathing, tai chi, relaxation and meditation, and other sorts of physical exercise. At first you will need active support to learn how to relax – letting go of tension is another habit we have to break. Relaxation is like changing the idling speed on a car. When a car engine turns over too quickly, wasting precious fuel and putting strain on the engine, a mechanic can reset the idling speed at a much lower level. Similarly, when stress, worry and perpetual hurry have speeded us up too much, making us tense, irritable and inefficient, we can learn how to let go and attain a much calmer, gentler state of being.

As with changing the way we deal with our emotions, it can be difficult to learn to relax on our own. It may be necessary at first to be relaxed passively by someone else. This can be achieved through a massage, aromatherapy or reflexology sessions, or by going for spiritual healing. Once you begin to get the feeling of what it is like to be relaxed, this can be built upon at home with the use of relaxation tapes or CDs or by learning relaxation techniques directly from a relaxation therapist. An alternative is to attend relaxation, yoga or tai chi classes. The beauty of yoga and tai chi, which both come from the East, is that they combine physical exercise with relaxation, breathing and meditation exercises. These techniques are specifically designed to simultaneously strengthen the body and calm the mind and nervous system. This is exactly what is needed for most smokers, whose nervous systems get progressively more jangled as they continue to smoke. Achieving optimal physical and mental health will be dealt with fully in Chapter 4, and contacts for counselling, relaxation, yoga, tai chi and meditation classes can all be found in Appendix 1.

The social aspects of smoking

Another part of giving up smoking is breaking the reflex action of smoking at the end of meals, with alcohol (either at home or in pubs and restaurants), after difficult jobs, or at certain times during your day. To overcome these habits, you must first identify what triggers them and then try to form a strategy to change your behaviour at these key points.

The most common trigger point for most smokers is the end of a meal. Try to find something else to do at your trigger points to replace having a cigarette. For example, if you are at home you could lie down and listen to a ten-minute relaxation tape instead of having a cigarette. You could go outside and get some fresh air in the garden if you have one, or take a walk around the block. It may be a good time to read or even take a nap. At work you will have to be more creative, but it may still be possible to sit quietly for a few minutes and do a relaxation exercise – even if this is in the loo!

If your trigger is drinking alcohol at social or business meetings, finding replacement tactics is obviously much harder. In fact, this is usually the time when people's good resolutions crumble and those who have successfully given up for a few days lapse into smoking again. If this is a vulnerable moment for you, then it may be wise to avoid alcohol and your usual social meetings while you are giving up smoking. It may even be a good idea to avoid going to restaurants, bars, pubs and clubs where you know you will be severely tempted, until you have stopped smoking altogether for around six weeks.

Quite often by this point newly reformed non-smokers find smoky atmospheres really hard to cope with. This is because the cleansing mechanisms in their lungs and windpipe are coming back to life again, and the irritation and unpleasant taste and smell of smoke become really noticeable and hard to take. It is a good sign when this starts to happens because it shows the body is beginning to recover from smoking. It will also serve to strengthen your resolve to give up long term.

In terms of passive smoking, pubs and clubs are the worst place to be as literally hundreds of people can be crowded together smoking in a very confined space, often with grossly inadequate ventilation. Passive smoking is in fact classed as an occupational cancer risk for bar staff, and there is a desperate need in society for non-smoking pubs and clubs. Try to avoid smoky places if you can or complain regularly and vociferously to the owners or even to the local Department of the Environment if you think there is a health risk being caused by inadequate ventilation.

Therapeutic help
Many people have found hypnosis or self-hypnosis useful

to help them overcome smoking cravings or reflex smoking in response to key triggers. The hypnotist will try to help smokers break their smoking patterns, replacing this self-destructive behaviour with positive thoughts and feelings. Another form of therapeutic help which has proven effective is acupuncture. The acupuncturist uses pressure points to liberate chemicals called endorphins – neuropeptides in the brain which can give us a feeling of satisfaction that helps to reduce the urge to smoke.

It is also a good idea to plan for a regular weekly or twice-weekly massage during the first six weeks of giving up to relax you. The expense of this can be justified on the basis of the money you are saving by not smoking!

It would also be helpful whilst giving up to take:

- 1000 mg of vitamin C three times a day

- 50 mg of B complex a day a day

- 100 mg of zinc orotate a day

These vitamins and minerals will:

- help repair lung tissue damage caused long term by smoking (particularly zinc).

- boost the immune system and protect against infections (particularly vitamin C). When smoking stops, the lungs temporarily start to secrete more mucus. This can make people prone to infections such as bronchitis or even pneumonia.

- help calm the nervous system (particularly vitamin B).

But even with the support of all the approaches mentioned above, the most important thing is the intention to stop.

Forming the intention to stop smoking
It may sound like an obvious thing to say, but the more you want to stop smoking, the easier it will be and the more likely you are to succeed. So, if you are a smoker take time right now to think about how important it is to stop smoking.

With a pen and a piece of paper, answer the following questions:

- Why do you want to give up smoking?

- What does smoking give you?

- What will make it difficult for you to give up smoking?

- How can you replace the benefits you get from smoking in a healthy way?

- How chemically dependent are you on cigarettes?

- Will you require help with nicotine replacement to stop?

- How emotionally dependent are you on cigarettes?

- What level of emotional support will you need to give up smoking?

- What could you do instead of smoking at your normal 'trigger points' to avoid having a cigarette?

Look at your answers and decide whether you are really ready to give up smoking. Once you have decided you are ready to make the commitment to yourself, take a fresh piece of paper and write down a large and clear statement of intention for yourself. This could be 'I choose to give up smoking now' or 'I will give up smoking now' or 'I will successfully give up smoking now' – whichever feels the most comfortable to you.

Then, make a second statement, listing all the support you will need – be it a counsellor, relaxation therapist, hypnotherapist, acupuncturist, masseur, support group, 'stop smoking' agency, doctor or nicotine patches.

Third, write down the people you will ask to support you in giving up smoking. It is important to consciously enrol partners, key family members, colleagues and friends to help you in case the going gets tough during the first few weeks. Tell them your intention so they can serve as witnesses to this commitment. Explain to them exactly the type of help you will need, and how they may best support you. This may be anything from asking them not to smoke in front of you, offer you cigarettes or confront you if possible if there are problems during the first six weeks, to asking them to be extremely kind and patient with you. Or you can simply explain that you will not be socializing as normal until you have beaten the habit. You may also want to tell them how you want them to react if they see you smoking!

The advice is then to repeat to yourself every single day your commitment to stop until you are well and truly clear of your smoking habit. You may want to stick up your written intention in a prominent place in the house or at work, but actually saying it to yourself each day and visualizing yourself as a non-smoker is a very powerful thing to do.

Another thing you can do is save the money you would have spent on cigarettes to reward yourself, perhaps something for your wardrobe or home, or a lovely holiday or some other treat.

The importance of giving up smoking cannot be stressed enough. The benefits will have repercussions in every area of your life, making you feel much better, happier and fitter within just a few weeks of stopping.

Alcohol

When Angela Burns was diagnosed with breast cancer, it forced her to re-evaluate her life. She was a professional woman, working as a manager with a large international retail organization, and liked to work hard and play hard. She is the first to admit that this meant drinking heavily on a regular basis. Angela was first diagnosed with breast cancer in 1991, when a mammogram picked up an early tumour in one of her breasts. She had a lumpectomy and radiotherapy and went back to work and her old lifestyle without a second thought.

It was only when she was diagnosed with a second lump in the same breast in 1995, for which she needed a mastectomy, that Angela realized she needed to start thinking about making some serious changes to her life. During rest and recuperation after the operation, she became aware for the first time in her working life of just how tired she was. She also had huge regrets about not taking action after the first diagnosis.

A doctor suggested she looked at what was on offer at the Bristol Cancer Help Centre and Angela joined the residential week-long course. Since then, Angela has made lots of changes to her life. Psychologically, she discovered she was not looking after herself properly and was always putting her team at work and other members of the family before herself. Energy wise, she had run her batteries completely flat because of her fast lifestyle. Despite her doubts about spiritual healing, she tried it, and now finds it both wonderfully calming and energizing. She also uses reflexology and relaxation techniques.

Angela stopped drinking alcohol every day, saving a drink for the weekends, and cut out spirits completely. She switched to goat's and sheep's cheese initially, and has now cut dairy products out of her diet altogether. She has a little fish and chicken but has stopped eating salt, smoked foods, red meat, pre-prepared foods like pâtés and pork pies, and doesn't drink coffee. Angela is now on a low-fat diet, eating organic fruit and vegetables wherever possible. All this doesn't mean that she has become completely puritanical though. She does indulge in fish and chips and a pint of beer every now and again!

The biggest change was that Angela decided to reduce her stress dramatically and relinquish her demanding job, retiring at the age of fifty. Doing this meant that it was far easier to seriously reduce her intake of alcohol once she no longer 'needed' it to manage her stress. She now does a part-time week with an enjoyable variety of paid and voluntary work mixed with plenty of gentle, fun, creative projects. Five years after secondary diagnosis she is feeling fine and looks radiant. Her new motto is to do all things in moderation, and her new game plan is to drink one bottle of champagne a week rather than seven bottles of plonk!

Changing your use of alcohol

Two units of alcohol a day for women and three for men are the recommended safe levels. (One unit of alcohol is equal to a small glass of wine, half a pint of beer or a pub measure of spirits.) Women who regularly consume three units a day and men four units incur progressive risk to their health, including an increased risk of cancer. Alcohol increases the risk of cancers of the mouth, throat, larynx (voice box), oesophagus (gullet), liver and breast, and the risk goes up as consumption increases. People who smoke as well as drink alcohol over the safe limit are at a considerably higher risk.

Even when staying within the recommended daily amounts, there is a good chance a person can become dependent on alcohol. As with smoking, alcohol dependence can be chemical and emotional. If you have become fixed in a pattern of regular drinking or actively need a drink at specific times of the day or during social situations, it is time to look seriously at why you are dependent on alcohol and then maybe start to find healthier ways of meeting the needs you are currently fulfilling with a drink.

Alcohol and its by-products are very toxic to the body, causing premature ageing, gut and liver disease, diseases of the nervous system and cardiovascular problems.

Heavy drinking increases the risk of certain cancers and can cause social and emotional distress. Alcohol, smoking and stress are currently the biggest thieves of vitality and health in Western society. Of course, these things go hand in hand, since stress increases our urge to drink and smoking increases too.

Ideally, it is best to stop drinking on a daily basis altogether. There should be gaps of at least two to three days between drinking alcohol to give the body a chance to detoxify and literally heal up again after an intake of alcohol. People who drink regularly get used to the effects of alcohol and are less sensitive to how toxic it is making them. But as anybody who drinks intermittently knows, it takes at least two days to feel fully recovered after an evening of drinking three or more units of alcohol. Try to make alcohol something just for special times and think twice before routinely having an alcoholic drink at social gatherings, business lunches or when you get home from work.

Chemical dependency

If you are 'hooked' on alcohol and literally need a drink to stop feeling bad physically – to stop shaking or feeling sick – you may need medical help to be weaned off it. Medication is available which is much less addictive than alcohol and helps to calm the mind while the body gets used to alcohol withdrawal. Unlike nicotine replacement therapy, this cannot be bought over the counter and you will need the help of a doctor or psychiatrist to take this route. You may even need a few days in hospital or a treatment centre to help you through the withdrawal period because long-term heavy drinking can leave you feeling pretty rough physically and psychologically when you stop. However, once through this difficult period you will start to feel better than you have for ages. Ask yourself 'Am I sick and tired of feeling sick and tired?' and resolve to become free of alcohol dependence. Alcohol is a seriously nasty drug, and the sooner you can get off it the better.

Emotional dependency

As with cigarettes, there is a big problem with emotional dependency on alcohol. Although alcohol is used to cover up feelings of anxiety, insecurity and poor self-esteem, regular use of it in fact makes a person's mental state far worse. People who drink excessive amounts of alcohol tend to be aggressive and violent and have heightened feelings of guilt and remorse. In general, thinking processes are slowed down, and with continued heavy alcohol use the damage to the nervous system can be catastrophic, with severe memory loss and impaired sensation and muscle function in the limbs.

Because excessive alcohol consumption causes such a vicious cycle of psychological problems, it is often an enormous task to rebuild emotional health and gain a strong positive self-image after a long period of alcohol abuse. Once you recognize any of the signs of alcohol dependency it is therefore important to nip these in the bud before you get on to the slippery slope of full-blown alcoholism. If you think you are an alcoholic, or seriously alcohol dependent, the best known and most effective way of getting support is through Alcoholics Anonymous. Their famous and very effective 'twelve-step programme' helps people to let go of alcohol and thus free themselves from the behaviour and attitudes of mind which accompany their drinking, replacing them with healthier coping strategies. If your drinking is not heavy enough to merit this level of intervention but you still recognize you are somewhat psychologically dependent on alcohol, then it would be wise to follow the advice given earlier for giving up smoking: go to a counsellor, join a support group, and learn to develop inner strength through the use of complementary therapies and self-help techniques. You will then be able to develop healthier ways of getting your emotional needs met.

What makes alcohol so popular is its power to relax and disinhibit. In the early stages of intoxication, people feel a lift in their emotional state. But this turns into a depressant effect after around three units. It is very easy, however, to learn how to achieve a deep state of relaxation naturally by learning relaxation and meditation techniques. Once you master these techniques you can use them when you would normally reach for a drink. When you first get home from work is a good time to employ such a technique, because often that one drink to relax you turns into two, three or more. This more than likely results in a very non-productive, uncreative evening, and one which will leave you hungover and far less able to work well the next day.

By contrast, half an hour of relaxation or meditation will allow the tension and exhaustion of the day to melt away, leaving you refreshed, open and receptive and able to have a far more constructive and creative time. In fact, people who meditate regularly become progessively calmer and their desire for alcohol diminishes greatly. Once a meditation technique is established, alcohol becomes less and less desirable anyway, because the states of mind reached through meditation are so much more pleasant and exciting than those reached with alcohol.

If you need alcohol because you feel shy on a date or before getting intimate with your partner, again it is far, far better to learn to relax and develop communication skills than use drink as a social lubricant. Once you have got to know a new partner, relaxing together using relaxation techniques and massage with beautiful oils in candle light will result in a far more pleasurable and richer experience than if you had both got drunk! As for the lift given by alcohol, this is very brief and is quickly replaced with a depression of all the senses. There are many other ways of becoming excited and happier which do not involve feeling sick and ill the next day! If you do need alcohol to get through social situations, you may well need counselling or assertiveness training to help build your confidence. Another option is a massage course to build up your physical confidence and repertoire of social skills.

The social side of alcohol

Perhaps even more than with smoking, people automatically pick up a drink in response to social cues, irrespective of whether they have any desire for an alcoholic drink. Also, from a very young age, within our society we become hard-wired to feel that unless we get drunk we have not had a good time. Drinking can become competitive in some social circles with people trying to outdo each other in terms of alcohol consumption. Others with a more compulsive personality will just keep drinking, in the same way that some people will just keep eating, whether they really want to or not. For all these reasons and many more, we drink far too much alcohol in very unthinking, indiscriminate ways. Therefore, it is vital for our health to think about how we want to drink and to get back in control of our drinking habits.

Without doubt, nothing compares to an exquisite bottle of wine to accompany a good meal, a beautiful bottle of champagne to celebrate a special occasion, or a glass of really cold beer on a hot summer's day. These are some of the very great pleasures in life. The advice is the same as that given for red meat – replace quantity with quality. In this case drink smaller quantities of excellent (preferably organic) alcohol at special times rather than large quantities of inferior alcohol all the time as a form of socially acceptable valium!

To start new drinking habits, it may be wise, as with when you stop smoking, to break your normal social routine, giving the pubs or clubs you usually go to a miss until you have had a chance to re-orientate yourself. You may need to take this even further if it is going to be impossible to go back to these places without overdrinking. If this is the case, you may need to consider a more radical change, replacing evenings normally spent in the pub with other things like exercise, evening classes or creative, self-expressive projects which will probably bring you far more satisfaction in the long run. You could also spend this time getting closer to those you love or taking time to be on your own.

There is of course the theory that a glass of wine a day actually protects against coronary heart disease and heart attacks. This is probably due to two factors. Firstly, plant nutrients in grapes include important vitamins, minerals, enzymes and other phytochemicals. Secondly, alcohol has a relaxing effect. However, both of these effects can be achieved in non-toxic ways – the first by eating fruit, vegetables and, of course grapes; the second by learning and practising relaxation. Overall it must surely be better to avoid the toxic effects of alcohol and get the benefits in safe, healthy ways through good diet and relaxation.

Hopefully, over time, if more and more adults change their drinking habits a new attitude to alcohol will pass down through the generations and we will begin to see a reduction in the terrible suffering caused by excessive use of this very toxic drug.

So, in summary, healthy use of alcohol involves:

- avoiding drinking alcohol every day.

- drinking no more than three units for a woman and four units for a man at any one time.

- recognizing and meeting emotional needs in healthy ways rather than by using alcohol.

- seeking medical and psychological help if addicted to alcohol.

Hormone replacement therapy and the pill

HRT

The conventional medical opinion is that the risks of hormone replacement therapy are outweighed by its protective effects, such as preventing osteoporosis. However, knowing that many cancers, particularly breast cancers, are hormonally sensitive makes me extremely worried about the use of HRT. My own advice is to avoid taking oestrogen-based or oestrogen progesterone combined HRT altogether unless there is a medical reason (such as osteoporosis) to do so. If vaginal soreness or dryness is a problem after menopause, you can use oestrogen cream or pessaries which can be obtained from your doctor. Where a low bone density has been diagnosed and osteoporosis seems likely, or there is a strong family history of osteoporosis, it is then up to each individual to make an informed choice based on her own circumstances and age.

Progesterone HRT

A new trend is to give progesterone-only HRT, which is considered a safer option. This is because progesterone is thought to be less of a stimulatory hormone than oestrogen. However, because some breast tumours are also progesterone receptor positive, it would seem unwise at present to prescribe progesterone-only HRT on a wide scale until more is understood. My advice therefore is to avoid taking HRT altogether, relying on a healthy and fulfilling lifestyle with good diet and exercise to maintain health and beauty after the menopause.

The skin of the body can be kept beautiful with oils and body creams, as can the skin of the face. Taking regular vitamin E and flax seed oils, and using facial creams containing retin A will also help keep the face looking good. Hot flushes are helped by vitamin E and flax seed oil, and herbal preparations such as agnus castus, black cohosh and 'Menopausal Herb Formula' (see Appendix 1) can help to smooth a woman's passage through the menopause. Many women find reflexology helps to ease the hormonal transition, because both the pituitary gland and the ovaries can be stimulated through reflexes in the feet.

The pill
Advice on the Pill in relation to cancer is harder. The conventional medical view is that because the risks of the Pill stop when a woman comes off it, and because in general the Pill is taken by women under the age of forty-five in whom the risk of breast cancer is much lower, the benefits outweigh the risks. This is all very well but increasing numbers of young women are getting breast cancer and the disease is often more virulent because of the high levels of circulating oestrogen. It is therefore better for women to use an alternative to the Pill as soon as other forms of contraception are suitable for them. However, during the early years of sexual activity, the benefits of the Pill still probably outweigh the risks. Thereafter, it would be much better to use barrier methods such as the cap, condoms or an intrauterine device (IUD). Generally, an IUD is only recommended for women who have had children. It must also be remembered that the coil and cap do not protect against

infectious diseases which can cause AIDS and cervical cancer. So unless you are in a steady relationship with someone who has been confirmed as infection free, condom use is vital.

Infections

The main hope of preventing cancer is by controlling infections such as HPV (human papillomavirus) and HIV, the two hepatitis viruses (B and C), herpes simplex and the viruses which cause lymphomas in Africa (which are linked with malarial disease). Prevention of HPV, HIV and hepatitis B can be achieved by having safe sex. It is important for everyone to maintain good sexual hygiene with new partners; it is even more important for those practising anal sex, where the likelihood of trauma and infection through blood contact is higher.

For those who know they are carrying these viruses, absolute integrity in terms of their sexual practice is essential, and they need to inform all potential partners of their health status. This will allow new partners to make informed choices about what sort of sexual activity they wish to get involved in before putting themselves at risk.

Work is continuing on vaccinations against all these viruses and it is likely that within our lifetimes such vaccines will be developed to protect people who are vulnerable. Vaccinations are already available against hepatitis B and C, and in some developing countries, where these viruses are more prevalent, vaccination programmes are already under way. It is possible to be vaccinated against hepatitis B and C in the UK if you believe yourself to be at risk, either through travel or because you have an infected partner.

Sunlight

For years, deeply tanned skin has been considered the pinnacle of health, beauty and sexiness. Now we face messages from the cancer research charities telling us there is actually no such thing as a safe and healthy tan.

We all crave sunshine and, indeed, become ill without it. We need sunshine on our skin to create vitamin D, which keeps our bones healthy. Without enough sunlight, we can also develop Seasonal Affective Disorder (SAD), which is a form of depression. However, in order to stay safe in the sun the advice is:

- avoid exposing the skin between 11 a.m. and 3 p.m.

- cover the skin with loose cotton clothes, a sun hat and sun glasses.

- take care not to burn the skin, being particularly careful if there is a cool breeze or light cloud.

- wear a sun screen of at least SPF 15 (see below) and a 4-star UVA rating.

- protect yourself when swimming as you can still get sunburnt in shallow water.

- look out for the new solar UV index on television weather forecasts at home and abroad.

- be extra sure to protect children, and keep babies under twelve months out of the sun completely.

- take extra special care if you have fair skin, blonde or red hair, and freckles because your type of skin burns more easily than most.

Do not make the mistake of thinking that it won't matter if you only go in the sun for two weeks on holiday. It is even more important to protect yourself if you get a sudden burst of intense sunshine in this way. It is also untrue that a tan from a sunbed will prepare you for tanning abroad. Sunbeds are based on UVA light rather than the UVB light from the sun's rays which burns the skin. People with dark or black skins do not burn as easily as those with fair skins, but it is still possible for black and Asian people to get sunburnt.

The SPF (sun protection factor) on a sunscreen gives an indication of how long you can stay in the sun without burning. For example, if you normally burn in ten minutes, wearing an SPF of 15 will protect you for fifteen times longer, i.e. for two and a half hours. However, after two and a half hours, no additional amounts of sunscreen will stop you from burning. A big problem is that sunscreens are often applied too thinly and can be rubbed or washed off. So, during this two-and-a-half-hour period, it is important to reapply cream to ensure its effectiveness. Thereafter, it is essential to cover up with loose clothing and a sun hat, or to sit in the shade. Some people worry about whether they will get sunburnt through glass. This is very unlikely, but it is possible to be exposed to some UVA rays as these can pass through glass. You are most at risk if you have:

- a tendency to burn easily and tan with difficulty.

- had skin cancer.

- a large number of moles.

- sun spots, which are a warning sign the skin has had too much exposure to the sun and is more prone to skin cancer.

It is also recommended that you do not use sunbeds to achieve a tan. These work mainly by giving UVA radiation to the skin which, whilst not burning the skin, is thought to play a potential role in the development of skin cancer. It is much safer to use tanning milks and creams to achieve a tanned look.

Electromagnetic radiation

The most obvious sources of concern about electromagnetic radiation in everyday life are mobile phones, microwave ovens, computers, electric pylons and office environments where strong electromagnetic fields may be set up by large amounts of electrical and electronic equipment.

Mobile phones
The advice is to keep use of mobile phones to a minimum and to use those with ear and mouth piece attachments (hands-free sets) rather than those that have to be held to the head. Mobile phones can also be kept in protective casing, and devices are also available to keep emissions to an absolute minimum (see Appendix 1).

Microwave ovens

For nutritional reasons (see page 58), the use of microwave ovens should ideally be avoided. If you do use a microwave, follow the instructions to the letter, strictly observing standing times for food. Make sure you are not using old or faulty equipment which may be leaking microwaves into the kitchen.

Computers

Always use a protective screen in front of your computer terminal to protect yourself against radiation. Take regular breaks from computer work. Do not leave your computer on if it is not in use. Try to avoid jobs that involve sitting in front of a computer all day every day.

Electricity

Living or keeping animals close to electric pylons is not advisable because these structures emit strong electrical fields and positive ions and radioactive particles towards them. It is also unhealthy to live over heavy-duty electrical cabling or near large electrical terminal points. Working in electric power stations may also be risky.

At work, it is up to your employer to ensure exposure levels are safe. If you are concerned, ask your employer to have the levels checked. Of particular concern at work and home are extra-low-frequency electromagnetic fields which have been specifically associated with cancer. Keep electrical equipment turned off when not in use and do not sleep with an electric blanket switched on. If you have any concerns about the levels of electromagnetic radiation around your home or place of work, seek advice from the local Electricity Board or Department of the Environment.

Radioactivity

Naturally occurring radioactivity is linked to the presence of radon gas. You can find out from your local Department of the Environment whether you live in an area with high radon gas levels. If you do, you can ask to have your premises checked for gas levels and, if necessary, build in protective materials or move. If you live close to either nuclear power stations or radioactive dumping sites, it is also advisable to get the Department of the Environment to check background radiation levels. Don't forget, their job is to protect you! The more the public takes an interest in these matters, ultimately the safer we will all be.

If you work around radioactive materials be extremely careful with their use and wear full protective clothing at all times.

Earth energies

Knowing what earth energies affect your home is very interesting, and advisable. A dowser can tell you what electromagnetic fields and currents are affecting your property and how best to position beds and other furniture to minimize the negative effects of these energies. If you are considering building a house or property, get your plot assessed first so that you can build in an optimum location.

Environmental pollution

Carcinogens in the home

It is important to try to eliminate all carcinogenic chemicals from the home environment. If it is at all possible, declare your home a no-smoking area. Refer to the list in Appendix 2 of all the household products which can contain carcinogens and see if you can avoid their use. To be absolutely sure which brands contain the offending chemicals, get hold of a copy of the *Safe Shopper's Bible*. You can then select brands which are completely carcinogen free.

Occupational carcinogens

Chemical carcinogens

It is vital to ensure you are not exposed to chemical carcinogens at work. Check the table of occupational hazards in Chapter 1, and check with the appropriate department at work to ensure you are being adequately protected. All places where dangerous chemicals are used should have proper safety measures in place, including the wearing of protective clothing and the use of protective handling equipment. As mentioned earlier, if you are self-employed and using dangerous chemicals (for example, farmers, artists and those in the building trade) you must be just as rigorous about safety measures as those working in a more closely monitored industrial environment.

Radiation

If you work as a radiologist or radiographer, or in any of the nuclear fuel or power industries, it is vital to keep a very accurate check of your levels of radiation exposure.

Medical causes

There are many medical causes of cancer, as discussed in Chapter 1. These usually stem from the use of diagnostic electromagnetic radiation or from medicines and procedures used to treat medical conditions. Make sure medical testing is always kept to a minimum. When accepting medical treatments of any sort make sure you are aware of all the side-effects so that you can make a properly informed choice about whether or not you wish to take the risks involved.

CHAPTER 3: EARLY DETECTION OF CANCER

The seriousness of a cancer diagnosis can be reduced greatly if it is made early. It is therefore advisable to know the early warning symptoms of cancer and how to check yourself and get the necessary medical screening.

EARLY SYMPTOMS

Symptoms to look out for which could indicate cancer include:

- a new or unusual lump anywhere on the body or in the abdomen

- a change in the appearance of a mole, or a sore on the skin or in the mouth that won't heal

- persistent coughing, hoarseness, or blood in the sputum

- prolonged constipation or diarrhoea, or blood in the stool

- difficulty in passing urine, or blood in the urine

- unexplained weight loss

- unexplained fatigue

- difficulty swallowing and unexplained nausea

- severe headaches and odd neurological symptoms (i.e. malfunctions in the nervous system such as weakness or numbness)

- unexplained abdominal swelling

- vaginal bleeding between periods, and any vaginal bleeding after the menopause

Of course, all these symptoms can occur as a result of conditions much less serious than cancer and, more often than not, a doctor will be able to reassure you that nothing is seriously wrong. However, it is important not to be reassured too easily until all the appropriate tests have been done. All too often, GPs give reassurance on the basis of a clinical examination in the surgery, only to be proved wrong at a later date. GPs expect patients to come back if symptoms persist, so it is very important to trust yourself and keep going back if you think something is not right. Far too many people go to their GP over and over again before they get sent for appropriate X-rays, blood tests or other investigations, only to discover in the end that a cancer which could have been treated easily as a primary has now developed secondary spread. If you are concerned your GP is not responding appropriately, get a second opinion from another GP or even arrange to get investigations done privately.

Lumps and bumps

The usual medical response to the presentation of an unusual lump or bump is to biopsy it in order to make a histological diagnosis of the tissue within the lesion. This involves taking a sample of the lump with a needle or cutting a little bit of the lump out and sending it to a laboratory to be looked at under the microscope. A biopsy lets doctors know whether the lump is a cancer or not and if they need to look for other areas of disease within the body. Some controversy surrounds the practice of doing biopsies. If possible, it is better to have a lump removed altogether than have it biopsied because, if the lump is cancerous, there is a risk that cancer cells will spread along the track of the biopsy needle or the line of the incision. While it is more trouble for a doctor or consultant to remove a lump in its entirety, this procedure is safer, if it can be arranged.

The other option is to have either an ultrasound, CT or MRI scan. These tests are often used anyway if the lump is deep within the body, and today with the very high-level diagnostic skills available, it is often possible to diagnose cancer in these far less invasive ways.

So, if a lump of any sort appears on or underneath the skin, ask for it to be removed completely for analysis. If a lump appears in the breast, ask for it to be investigated first with ultrasound and/or mammography rather than a biopsy. If suspicion is high that this is cancer, it is wise then to proceed straight to a lumpectomy. This means removing the entire lump, including enough healthy breast tissue to be sure that the lump has been taken cleanly from the breast.

Lumps or bumps in the abdomen are also investigated by scans or ultrasound. Again, if suspicion is high, these can be removed either during a laparoscopy, where a tiny keyhole incision is made in the abdomen or, if more serious, during investigative abdominal surgery.

Changes to the skin and mouth

If changes to the skin develop, you should see a dermatologist (skin specialist). Sores in the mouth that will not heal need the attention of either a dentist or an ear, nose and throat (ENT) surgeon. Again, if it is possible to avoid a biopsy and move straight to complete excision of the lesion, this is preferable. Usually, dermatologists, dentists and ENT specialists can tell by looking at these conditions whether they are cancerous or not, and are likely to go straight to excision rather than biopsy.

Coughing, hoarseness, and blood in the sputum

This is one of the areas where a cancer diagnosis is far easier to miss. Many people suffer each year from colds, coughs and chronic lung diseases such as bronchitis, bronchiectasis and occupational lung disease, and most of us will have a sore throat at least once a year. Usually smokers have some soreness and hoarseness in the throat area all the time, and so it is understandable that GPs do not send everyone with these symptoms for scans and X-rays.

Persistent blood in the sputum should definitely be taken seriously by doctors. Sometimes, a very sudden show of blood in the sputum which never re-appears is caused by the rupturing of a small blood vessel in the lungs during heavy coughing. But if bleeding continues it is much more likely to be from an area of ulceration in the windpipe (bronchus) or lungs, which could easily be due to cancer. People with persistent hoarseness should be sent to an ENT specialist. Blood in the sputum should be checked out with a bronchoscopy investigation. This involves a doctor looking directly at the windpipe and lungs whilst the patient is under sedation to see if there are any growths or areas of ulceration.

Persistent coughing merits a chest X-ray and sputum test, and may also require a bronchoscopy. A sputum test can identify not only cancer cells, but also infectious agents and the presence of blood, and sputum samples are sent to three different parts of the pathology department. So, if you are concerned, ask your GP whether the sputum has been checked specifically for cancer cells.

Change in bowel habit

Again, this is a very difficult area for GPs to assess, as constipation, diarrhoea and even blood in the stool are very common. The most common cause of blood in the stool is piles, which is caused by prolonged tightness of the anal sphincter muscle. Another explanation is anal fissures or fistulas, which are cracks in the skin of the anus. When you have piles, fissures or fistulas, you tend to know all about them because they make passing a motion very painful. Therefore, people are likely to know whether blood in the stool is caused by these sorts of problems.

Crohn's disease and ulcerative colitis are other relatively common causes of blood in stools. And, as before, people with these illnesses tend to know about them. Patients with these long-term problems have abdominal bloating, often a mixture of diarrhoea and constipation, and a combination of mucus and blood in the stool, whilst generally feeling unwell. These illnesses are intermittent and flare-ups are often closely related to periods of high anxiety or stress.

The diagnostic tests for these two conditions are similar to those used to detect bowel cancer. Usually, the doctor starts with a sigmoidoscopy, which involves looking directly into the first part of the bowel. If Crohn's disease or ulcerative colitis is present, the lining of the colon will look sore, red and inflamed. Sometimes, doctors need to look further into the bowel and this is done with a colonoscopy. During this investigation, the whole length of the large bowel can be viewed as far as the appendix (where the small bowel begins).

Exactly the same approach is likely to be employed if a doctor is trying to rule out bowel cancer. But, in addition, the patient may be given a barium enema followed by X-rays of the bowel so that any growths can be detected. These tests will rule out or confirm the presence of cancer in the large bowel. To see whether there is a tumour in the small bowel, a different test (called a barium swallow) and follow through is required. This is based on exactly the same principle, but the radio opaque material is swallowed rather than introduced into the body through the anus, as with a barium enema.

When a diagnosis of Crohn's disease, ulcerative colitis or polyps has been made there should be regular screening to look for bowel cancer because it is more common in people with these conditions than in those with normal bowels.

Persistant diarrhoea or unexplained constipation should also be checked as these too can be symptoms of cancer. More commonly, though, they are found to be due to 'irritable bowel syndrome', 'spastic colon' or just poor diet.

Urinary problems

Prostate cancer, where the enlarged gland presses on the urethra or out-flow tube from the bladder, can cause men to have difficulty passing urine. However, this symptom is very common, especially in older men. Mostly, it is caused by a benign growth of the prostate gland known as benign prostatic hypertrophy. Men who have difficulty passing urine are referred to a urologist, who will ascertain first if the prostate gland has grown and, second, whether the growth is benign or malignant. A blood test measuring levels of prostatic specific antigen (PSA) can help to establish the presence of prostate cancer. The doctor will then usually go on to perform a rectal ultrasound test during which it is customary to take needle biopsies which can be analysed under the microscope.

As previously mentioned, it is better to avoid biopsies if possible, and if cancer can be diagnosed through the PSA and rectal ultrasound scan alone, this is preferable. Difficulty passing urine in women should also be taken seriously, especially if it is painless. If there is pain, the bleeding is more likely to be caused by infection. But if not, there may well be a mass of some sort blocking the flow. In this case, the likely course of action would be a pelvic ultrasound.

Blood in the urine of both men and women should always be taken seriously. The most common cause is infection, but it can be caused by cancer in the kidney, ureter (tube from the kidney to the bladder), bladder or urethra (tube from the bladder to the outside). If infection has been ruled out or treated and bleeding still persists, the bladder can be examined directly by having a cystoscopy (visual examination of the bladder). The kidney, ureter and bladder can also be looked at by ultrasound investigation, or by injecting into a vein in the arm a dye which can then be seen on an X-ray of the abdomen, revealing any problems throughout the urinary tract.

Weight loss

If nothing else in your life has changed particularly, you are eating and exercising as usual and you suddenly lose a significant amount of weight, with no obvious explanation, this ought to be investigated. You should start to be concerned if you find you have lost between 3 and 6 kilos (7–14 pounds). Sudden weight loss can also occur due to emotional traumas such as bereavement or the break-up of a relationship, or alternatively the excitement at the beginning of a new one. Tummy bugs can also cause quite marked weight loss, as can a change in diet. For example, people who change from a high meat and fat diet to a vegan diet often lose a considerable amount of weight. Sudden weight loss may also occur if a new medication is started, such as a diuretic, which causes excess fluid to be passed out of the body in the urine.

If none of these situations apply, and weight loss has occurred for no obvious reason, it is best to get checked over by your GP. The doctor is likely to perform blood tests to look for cancers such as lymphoma and leukaemia. A liver function blood test will also show if there is cancer affecting the liver. If severe weight loss occurs, it is possible that there is already secondary cancer in the body affecting the liver or lungs. But weight loss may occur with primary bowel cancer that is affecting the normal bowel habit or making eating and absorbing food difficult. It is therefore likely that the GP will do a physical examination of the abdomen or send a patient for an ultrasound check of the abdominal organs to rule out the presence of cancers of the pancreas, liver, kidneys, ovaries or womb.

Fatigue

Fatigue as a symptom is even more non-specific and is linked to a whole range of health problems. In fact, Tired All The Time syndrome (TATT) is believed to be the most common problem currently presented in GP surgeries. In the general population, fatigue is usually the result of a combination of high stress, low exercise and poor diet, often aggravated by toxins from smoking and drinking. The next most common cause of fatigue is post-viral fatigue which can occur after a nasty virus infection. In some cases, this goes on to become full-blown ME (myalgic encephalomyelitis), causing extreme exhaustion and muscle weakness.

When fatigue is associated with cancer, it may be a sign of quite advanced disease. But many people with cancer say that, looking back, they had been feeling excessively tired for six months or even a year before being diagnosed. Fatigue should always be taken as a serious warning that all is not well and that it is time to take active steps to recover a healthy balance in life. Ways of doing this will be addressed fully in Chapter 4. However, if your fatigue does not fit with any obvious pattern or explainable cause, then a GP should assess you in the same way as for weight loss.

Difficulty in swallowing and nausea

If you have on-going difficulty swallowing which cannot be put down to a sore throat or laryngitis, you should get this investigated without delay. Difficulty swallowing or regurgitating food is often associated with a growth in the gullet or oesophagus, which must be treated as quickly as possible.

If eating often results in feeling nauseous, or if food just won't digest and keeps repeating on you, it is possible that the out-flow of food through the stomach or the small bowel is being impeded by a tumour. Once other causes of nausea – such as morning sickness, stomach upset, reaction to alcohol or drugs, and so on – have been eliminated, your GP is likely to refer you for an endoscopy to look directly at the gullet and stomach. If this is negative, it will probably be followed by a barium swallow and follow through and X-rays to look at the state of the small bowel.

If the bowel becomes completely obstructed by a tumour this will result in severe abdominal pain and vomiting, and this is treated as a medical emergency (see 'Unexplained Abdominal Swelling' below).

Headaches and neurological problems

Severe headaches are another nightmare area for GPs. The cause of a severe headache can range from a hangover or tension at one extreme, to meningitis or brain cancer at the other, both of which can be fatal. However, both of these conditions are relatively rare in comparison with the number of headaches which occur due to tension, migraine, hangovers, non-serious viruses or bacterial infections anywhere in the body, or for no apparent reason at all. This means a GP has to be pretty worried before referring someone for a scan to look for a brain tumour. It is therefore very important, if you have a strong suspicion that a headache is very odd, that you persist and convince your GP that you really are worried.

A GP will always act if there are accompanying neurological symptoms – signs indicating that the brain or other parts of the nervous system are malfunctioning in some way, such as when eyesight, hearing, balance, speech, smell, taste, muscle strength or sensation in any part of the body become affected. There may also be unexplained fits, vomiting, mental changes or even loss of consciousness. These symptoms will alert the GP that there could be something causing pressure in the brain that must be investigated immediately.

Unexplained abdominal swelling

If the abdomen has swollen up in an uncharacteristic way, a doctor will want to check that there are no big masses causing this problem. Abdominal masses can be caused by tumours in the womb, ovaries, bowel, liver and, occasionally, the pancreas or kidney, or by lymphoma. Masses in the abdomen are not always cancerous; they can be caused by large fibroids in the uterus, for example, which are completely benign. The other cause of abdominal swelling, which can be associated with cancer, is ascites. This is when the abdomen fills up with fluid, when the liver is diseased.

The abdomen can also swell for other non-cancerous

reasons, including gas accumulation, fluid retention and, of course, pregnancy! A doctor should first examine the abdomen, performing a vaginal or rectal examination as well, if necessary. If diagnosis is still unclear, the patient is likely to be referred for abdominal ultrasound or an abdominal X-ray. If there is any possibility of pregnancy, X-ray should be avoided in favour of ultrasound.

Sometimes, if the gut has become obstructed or blocked altogether, abdominal swelling is an emergency problem. In this situation, a person will suffer severe colicky pains and quite often nausea or vomiting, and it is best to go straight to casualty or ring for an ambulance or emergency GP. Obstruction can be caused by severe constipation at one extreme and cancer at the other, but must be treated quickly to avoid perforation of the bowel and peritonitis (which is infection of the abdominal cavity).

Vaginal bleeding

Most pre-menopausal women will have the odd bit of irregular bleeding between periods during their lifetime. However, persistent intermittent spotting between periods must be checked by a GP. Any bleeding at all after the menopause should be investigated straightaway too. Here, doctors will check for cancers of the vulva, vagina, cervix, endometrium (womb lining), womb or ovaries. Investigation may well start with a vaginal examination, which may proceed to a colposcopy. This gives a consultant gynaecologist a chance to have a good look at the cervix. If there are any abnormalities, it may then be necessary to take a sample of the womb lining in a procedure called a D and C (dilation and curettage). This may be backed up by ultrasound examination of the womb tubes and ovaries and/or laparoscopy, where the pelvic organs are looked at directly through a keyhole incision in the abdominal wall.

SELF-EXAMINATION

Self-examination for the symptoms of cancer is really an extension of getting to know your body and taking really good care of yourself in general. There are many areas of the body you cannot check yourself, but there are certainly some parts you can keep an eye on.

It is a very good idea to check your skin regularly. If possible, get a partner, family member or friend to check the areas that are not easy for you to see, perhaps while changing at a gym or swimming pool.

Get used to the normal consistency of your breasts; this applies to both males and females because, although rare, breast cancer can occur in men too. The advice is to check the four quadrants of the breast separately with a flat hand, sensing whether there are any lumps or bumps underneath the surface. It is also a good idea to stand in front of a mirror and raise your arms so you can look at the breasts from all angles to check for any dimpling, pulling or puckering of the skin. While you are doing this, you could feel the neck and underarm to check there is no obvious lymph gland swelling. From time to time, the groin can be checked in this way too, for signs which could alert you to problems in the abdomen or legs.

For men, it is a good idea to check the testicles regularly. Grip the scrotum in such a way that you immobilize the testicles and then feel each one all over its surface to make sure that all the contours are smooth and that you can feel no lumps and bumps. It is also a good idea to check your abdomen from time to time. Lie on your back with your knees bent and your feet flat on the floor or bed, then check the lower, mid and upper parts to make sure there are no lumps and masses within the abdominal cavity. However, be aware that if you are very constipated, this too can give the feeling that there are masses in the abdomen, but the reason for this should be fairly obvious to you.

Another good idea, especially if you are a smoker and drinker, is to look regularly within your mouth and at your lips to make sure there are no sores forming which do not appear to be healing.

SCREENING

Currently in the UK there is routine screening only for breast and cervical cancer. In addition, regular screening for colorectal cancer is carried out for certain people (see below), and often GPs or private health check-up clinics will do a PSA (prostate specific antigen) blood test on men over fifty to see if there is evidence of prostate abnormality. Other than this, it is really a question of being alert to symptoms which may appear or for abnormalities which may be found during self-examination. Above all, it is absolutely vital to trust your 'inner voice' or gut feeling if you sense something is really wrong with you, and get yourself tested appropriately until you're proved right or fully reassured.

Breast cancer

Screening for breast cancer is now routine for all women in the UK aged between fifty and sixty-five. An annual examination of the breasts by a doctor or nurse is also recommended for all women over forty. Women should go for a medical check-up immediately at any age if they find any change in the breast. Over the age of fifty, women in the UK are called for a routine mammogram, which is an X-ray examination of the breasts. This screening system is controversial and women's groups have lobbied for the age to be reduced to forty and extended to women aged sixty-five to seventy. Current calculations suggest that insufficient numbers of women under fifty would be picked up to justify the expense of this massive intervention. However, the Government has promised to extend breast screening to women aged sixty-five to seventy. This test can identify breast cancers before they can be found by self- or medical examinations.

Breast cancer screening is also controversial because of concern that repeated X-rays of the breasts may help contribute to cancer in those who do not have it. Many women prefer a combination of ultrasound screening and manual examination. But none of these three tests is foolproof: diagnosis has been missed with all three, and the risks of ultrasound are not yet fully understood either. There is definitely a need for safer methods of breast cancer screening to be developed which are more accurate, with less potential hazard.

If you have a strong family history of breast cancer, or a genetic susceptibility, then it is likely that you will be offered (or you should ask for) mammography from a much younger age. If you are invited to have a mammogram it is certainly advisable to take up the option because cancers which are detected in this way, before they are even palpable as a lump, are usually curable. This is because, at this early stage, spread has not usually occurred into the breast or neighbouring lymph nodes, and there are no accompanying metastases. If early breast cancers can be removed completely, then the chances of cure are very high.

Cervical cancer

After the breasts, the other part of the body that lends itself to routine screening is the cervix. Because cancer of the cervix affects both younger and older women, cervical screening goes on right through a woman's life, at regular three-yearly intervals in most areas of the UK. Again, it is wise to go for cervical screening because abnormalities in the cervix can be picked up even before they become cancerous. In this case, the lab report will say there are either viral changes or CIN (cervical intraepithelial neoplasia) 1, 2 or 3, and these changes should be taken seriously. Not everybody who has viral changes or

CIN will definitely get cancer, but at least 10 to 20 per cent of CIN 3 cervixes will become cancerous. If treated properly at this early stage, it is very unlikely there will be any further problem.

Colorectal cancer

These cancers are not routinely screened for within the UK. However, there is a case for regular screening if you have familial adenomatous polyposis or have one or more near relatives with colorectal cancer; if you have had a previous colorectal cancer yourself which has been removed; if you have a history of ulcerative colitis, Crohn's Disease or breast, uterine or ovarian cancer; or if you have had radiation treatment to the pelvis. Screening will involve rectal examination, testing for blood in the stools, sigmoidoscopy, colonoscopy and possibly a barium enema.

Genetic or 'family' cancers

Most cancers are not hereditary. Even when more than one case of cancer appears in a family, it is more often than not just sheer coincidence. However, occasionally people do inherit an extra risk of developing the disease.

Inherited gene defects can cause a small proportion of breast and ovarian cancers, through the BRCA2 and, more rarely, BRCA1 genes. About 10 per cent of bowel cancers are inherited and a further 1 per cent arise as a result of

inherited familial adenomatous polyposis, which is initially a benign condition but can become malignant.
Retinoblastoma – a form of childhood eye cancer – is
inherited in four out of ten cases, and melanoma can also
run in families. All these conditions can be screened for.

However, even if you have a family history of cancer,
your risk may not be as high as you think it is. Individual
risk depends a great deal on how old the people in your
family were when they were diagnosed and how closely
related they are to you. The younger a person is when
diagnosed, the more likely it is that the cancer is due to
a genetic predisposition.

In order to assess your risk of developing cancer, it is
necessary to build up a picture of your family tree, indicating all close relatives who have had a cancer. From this
information, a calculation of your risk can be made and
advice given on what screening might be appropriate.

If there is a form of cancer that seems to run in your
family, particularly if it tends to develop at a young age,
you should talk it over with your GP. You should discuss
whether you need to be referred for screening at your
nearest hospital or at an Imperial Cancer Research Fund
family cancer clinic where people at risk are identified,
counselled and screened (see Appendix 1).

CHAPTER 4: HOW TO REVOLUTIONIZE YOUR PHYSICAL HEALTH

GETTING THE BODY TO FIGHT BACK

The first three chapters have taken an in-depth look at cancer: how common it is, its causes, its risk factors, and how relatively ineffective medicine is at treating the disease – all of which make pretty alarming reading. It is now time to look at the positive side of the story. There are many factors which can protect against the development of cancer. Cancer prevention really comes down to understanding these factors and learning how to boost the body's ability to protect itself against cancer.

A famous comment by Louis Pasteur is relevant to cancer prevention. After a lifetime of studying bacteria and the course of infectious diseases he announced quite simply on his deathbed 'Le terrain est tous' (literally, 'the soil (or terrain) is everything'). What he meant by this was: 'yes, it is wonderful to have vaccinations to deal with infections, but it is actually a combination of the internal environment within the body and the external environment in which we find ourselves that determines our susceptibility to infection. Only by working with the "terrain" or environment can we hope to tackle infectious illness.' Pasteur turned out to be quite right. The two things that made the biggest difference to death rates from infectious diseases were the creation of proper sewerage systems and a rise in the nutritional standards of the general public. Vaccinations alone were never going to be the answer to the problem of widespread infectious disease within the population.

With cancer we have an identical situation. We will never eradicate cancer with medical treatment. However, governments and research institutes of the world seem to have missed this point. To date, billions of pounds and dollars have been poured into cancer causes and treatment, and only a tiny fraction of the total research budget has been put into cancer prevention and helping to change our personal or collective environments. At the moment, developed countries spend more than 90 per cent of cancer research budgets on cancer treatments and causes and only about 5 per cent on prevention, with the rest being spent on research into cancer care.

From reading so far you will realize that cancer is, in most cases, a preventable disease for which we know the main causes. But it will take a determined and concerted effort, and a much more responsible attitude by individuals and society as a whole, to tackle this problem head-on and change the cancer picture.

It is time to get active and revolutionize your health and life by embarking on the holistic approach to cancer prevention. The first step in this process is to learn how to take control of the key factors that affect health and resistance to disease. These key factors are:

- healthy eating and cooking

- vitamin, mineral and herbal supplements

- exercise

- dealing with stress, anxiety and overwork

- sleep, rest and relaxation

- maintaining high energy levels

- achieving peace of mind

To help you understand why these factors are so crucial to health, I will first give a full explanation of the holistic model of health and illness. This will clarify why it is so crucial to address health at all levels of body, mind and spirit in order to prevent cancer.

THE HOLISTIC APPROACH
TO HEALTH

The idea that our body's physical health is related to our state of mind, body, spirit and environment, has been around for centuries. However, with the advent of science and Newtonian physics, there was a distinct shift towards a model of medicine where the body was seen either like a machine with parts which could be fixed if broken down or like a collection of chemical mechanisms which could be controlled artificially with man-made chemicals. This approach, which reached its zenith in the late twentieth century, has been responsible for some astounding progress in medicine, bringing with it the possibilities of such things as hip replacements, cataract removal, organ transplants and the controlling of many diseases through medication.

However, since the 1960s there has been great dissatisfaction with the idea of treating only the symptoms of disease without addressing the underlying cause. There has been a strong resurgence of interest in the idea that mind, body and spirit are connected, and that each individual is in fact connected to the whole of life and therefore to all other individuals. During the 1960s and 1970s, these 'alternative' ideas were ridiculed and opposed by orthodox doctors. But during the 1980s and 1990s, hard scientific evidence emerged which has forced people to take seriously the holistic model of health and illness.

The key message of the holistic approach is that, far from being simply human machines made up of a complicated set of parts and chemicals, we are very complex beings and the functionings of our mind, body and spirit really do interact, profoundly affecting our health and well-being. For example, nutrition affects not only physical health but also IQ and mental state. Exercise can radically change our mood, while meditation (which calms the mind) has a profound affect on our heart, breathing and immune function. It has also been shown that spiritual healing changes the brain wave pattern from stressed beta activity into self-healing alpha activity, as well as raising the level of the immune 'natural killer' cells that are so crucial in the body's fight against cancer.

But perhaps most extraordinary is the effect of prayer – which in scientific trials has been shown to improve significantly the chances of survival after a heart attack – and the technique of visualization, which if used during chemotherapy can significantly extend the survival time of cancer patients. Visualization is a 'mind over matter' technique where, in their 'mind's eye', individuals literally see themselves getting well or having good outcomes from treatment. And when people with cancer are helped to express their feelings of anger, grief and disbelief in support groups, this too has been shown to positively affect survival. Early studies showed that people who demonstrated a positive 'fighting spirit' when diagnosed with cancer survived up to 60 per cent longer than those who collapsed and became 'helpless and hopeless'. More recently, studies of cancer patients have consistently shown that the prognosis is far worse for those who are depressed and helpless than for those who cope better mentally.

The mind–body connection

Understanding of the mind–body connection has shot forward during the last few years. From the 1950s to the 1970s there was only a very basic understanding of how stress and fear adversely affect body function. What was known was that stress or fear causes adrenaline to be secreted, which in turn prioritizes the functioning of the brain and muscles for the well-known 'fight or flight' response. This means that when we are frightened or stressed, activity in the body is diverted away from the 'housekeeping functions' such as digestion, absorption, growth, immune response, healing and repair. As a result we can be mentally clear and physically strong to fight off the current threat or danger, or run like hell!

This short-term stress response is highly advantageous to our survival. If you are being chased by a tiger, digesting your breakfast or warding off infection is not exactly your highest priority! But if stress becomes prolonged or chronic, it can have a disastrous effect on health as the vital 'housekeeping' functions become compromised long term. Most of us these days live our lives in such pronounced states of anxiety or fear, it is as if we are permanently being chased by a tiger – whether it be in the form of a bank manager, taxman or mortgage company!

In prolonged stress, there are high cortisol levels in the body as well as high adrenaline levels. Cortisol, the natural steroid secreted by the adrenal glands, helps us deal with challenging situations. High cortisol and adrenaline levels directly inhibit our immunity to disease and infection. This has been clearly demonstrated both in the laboratory and in real life. Stress has also been shown to have an adverse effect on blood pressure, cholesterol and fat levels in the blood; it is also associated with irritability and an increased dependence on cigarettes, alcohol and drugs, with all their attendant problems.

The understanding of this mechanism through the 1960s and 1970s explained why prolonged stress and high levels of fear are so deleterious to the body, but it did not explain why emotions affect our health so strongly. People started to ask 'Why does falling in love cause eczema or irritable bowel syndrome to clear up?' and 'How can an old person die within weeks of their spouse dying, when there is nothing apparently wrong with them?' Neither did it explain why visualization or mind-over-matter techniques can have such a profound effect on our physiology.

The real revolution in our understanding of the mind–body connection has come through the new scientific field of psychoneuroimmunology (PNI). This revolution started in the 1970s with the discovery, by Dr Candace Pert, of a receptor in the brain for a substance resembling morphine. Shortly after this, the substance itself was discovered, and named endorphin or enkephalin. The discovery of this naturally occurring opiate in the brain triggered the discovery of over 200 other tiny messenger chemicals. These substances were named neuropeptides or informational substances. It was quickly realized that these substances are secreted not only in the brain and nerve tissue but also in all the other parts of the body.

With this discovery, it became clear that the old model – of a brain and nervous system communicating only through neurotransmitters at the ends of the nerves – was completely out of date. It was replaced by a model in which all the tissues of the body are able to communicate with each other through informational substances. This new approach was based on the fact that receptors for these substances were found simultaneously in the brain and many other tissues of the body. The pathways of the neuropeptides were tracked and it was shown that there was a communication loop from the brain to the tissues and back again. And so the amazing discovery was made that the tissues were 'talking' to the brain just as much as the brain was 'talking' to the tissues! But more than this, it was now clear that the body's tissues could communicate with each other too.

This concept is so revolutionary, it has completely blown apart the idea of the body as five separate anatomical systems working more or less independently (as has been taught in medical schools for the whole of the last century!). In fact, communication between all the systems of the body is so complex, even trying to imagine it is difficult. Bearing in mind that computers work on a binary system of two digits, the whole of Western music is composed on a scale of twelve intervals, and the English language is based on twenty-six letters, a neuropeptide communication system with a minimum of 200 units provides more possible combinations than we could even begin to imagine.

In practice, different emotional states create certain patterns of neuropeptide secretion and these strongly affect tissue functioning within the body. When people are stressed, depressed, distressed and emotionally repressed long term, the most common response is severe depression of immune function too. This affects both the activity of individual immune cells and the number of circulating immune cells.

However, it is not just the immune system that is affected. Studies have shown that the red blood cells of people who are depressed and stressed carry less oxygen, and that a whole range of tissue functions changes according to our predominant state of mind. Scientists have not yet managed to work out exactly how the mind-over-matter techniques of visualization or affirmation affect tissue functions. But certainly, circulating blood cell levels have been shown to change in response to a person's visualization of them increasing, demonstrating clearly that these techniques have very real physical consequences.

So where does all this fit into preventing cancer? Studies to date, looking at whether there is a link between stress and distressing life events and cancer, have had conflicting results – some studies show definite links, others do not. What PNI scientists are now telling us is that it is not stress or distress per se which is the problem but how an individual reacts to it. A concept called 'personality hardiness' is used to describe people who respond to stress and difficult situations quite positively, seeing them as an exciting challenge and source of potential empowerment rather than succumbing to anxiety, fear and feelings of powerlessness.

Certainly, people who are depressed, isolated and socially disadvantaged have higher rates of cancer and die more quickly from cancer than those who are happy, affluent and well supported. This fits with the observation that people who become helpless and hopeless when they are diagnosed with cancer fare much worse than those with fighting spirit. From this evidence – and the studies which show that cancer patients who express their feelings in support groups live longer, and that visuali- zation can extend survival time – it becomes clear that state of mind has a great deal to do with the body's ability to defend itself against cancer.

This is not the same as saying psychological factors cause cancer, or saying that people are in any way to blame if they do get cancer. The bottom line is that the Western lifestyle is extremely stressful and those who are prone to feeling more anxious, helpless and hopeless or who have lost their way in life are likely to be more vul- nerable to serious illness, and at greater risk if they get one. But the most important thing to say straightaway is that these ways of reacting to life can be changed, through a combination of psychotherapy, support and self-help. How to go about doing this will be addressed fully in the next two chapters.

To be really well, the body's physical needs must be met too, by eating healthy food and taking food supple- ments, by enhancing our energy and vitality, by express- ing our sexuality and by getting enough exercise, rest and relaxation. Fulfilling these needs enables us to free our bodies from the effects of fear and stress. But most of all, we must achieve peace of mind, making sure we have the most lively immune system possible. To do this, the primary question we must address concerns our state of mind and spirit.

Achieving peace of mind

The study and practice of meditation is a direct approach to achieving peace of mind. Meditation really is the king of the self-help techniques; as well as having profound benefits for immune function, it calms and strengthens the cardiovascular, nervous, gastrointestinal and respiratory systems. Certainly, meditating will calm the emotions and lift a person's mood and spirit. It will also lead to clearer thinking and far more efficient and effective working. The other way to achieve peace of mind is to deal directly with the stress of our overcrowded lives. These approaches will be addressed in full later in this chapter. Sometimes, however, peace of mind can never be achieved unless the underlying state of our spirit is tackled head-on.

Freeing the spirit

If you have become dispirited, or your spirit has been crushed or broken by life due to a combination of disappointment, grief and frustration, or perhaps simply because you have not found a way to fully express yourself, this can have a very depressing or even devastating effect on the immune system. This explains how an elderly person can die within six weeks of losing their spouse, and clearly illustrates that when the will to live has gone, the physical body can very quickly give way.

Sadly, many people nowadays exist in an unfulfilled state, having very little sense of purpose or meaning in their lives and no real sources of spiritual nourishment or emotional well-being. Often people live their lives based on the expectations and demands of others, having very little excitement or passion to enliven and vitalize them. Certainly, in the field of holistic cancer medicine, it is clear that when people lose the will to live or have no exciting, creative focus for their energy, no medicine, orthodox or complementary, will get them well. On the other hand, if this sense of purpose and passion is rekindled, people rapidly get well from the 'inside out' as their immune system comes back to life.

To free the spirit, it is often necessary to work on several fronts simultaneously. To start with, it is very important to attend to our 'emotional hygiene'. Many of us tend to repress our feelings, holding on to anger, hurt, guilt, grief and disappointment. These emotions then literally sit in the body, affecting our posture, breathing and tissue functioning through PNI mechanisms, and weighing down or burdening our spirit.

Once you start to tune into these things, it is very easy to see the emotions other people are hanging on to. If you look closely at people, you will see that their body language, breathing pattern, eyes and facial expressions say it all! In holistic medicine, the saying is, 'what the mind represses the body expresses'. We literally 'embody' the feelings we can't let go of. Shedding old emotions and, more importantly, learning how to express rather than repress emotions, are crucial steps on the path towards good health.

The next step is identifying what drives your behaviour. Often, we are programmed from childhood to push ourselves relentlessly in order to prove ourselves; achieve success; win approval, love and affection; or achieve the perfection we think is expected of us. What this means is that, most of the time, we behave the way other people want us to be and our own unique spirit becomes submerged. Often, this is linked to low self-esteem and a tendency to take care of others while at the same time neglecting or abandoning ourselves. Once we have identified the slave driver, perfectionist, workaholic or approval-seeking sides of ourselves, the task is then to replace this programming with kinder, more encouraging and supportive messages which allow our real selves to emerge and flourish and our spirit to lift.

This brings us to another fundamental part of the holistic approach to health – the belief that healthy living and spiritual development revolve around having a healthy relationship with yourself, others, and the environment in which you live. It is staggering how many people put themselves at the very bottom of the list of people to care for. Most people look after their houses, cars and pets far better than they look after themselves! Getting the relationship with yourself right will provide a solid foundation for everything else. If you take time to listen and respond to your own needs, and gradually work towards being true to yourself, your life and health will be transformed beyond recognition.

To take this process further, the next step is to spend time in retreat, counselling, psychotherapy or supportive group work, or to simply quieten down and listen to your inner voice to discover what your own core values and needs really are. It is vitally important to be involved in things that express your true self and give you a sense of purpose and meaning. Over time, try to work towards getting yourself living in the right place in the right way, with a lifestyle, home and job that truly reflect who you are.

It is also important to ensure you can both express love and receive the love you need. This may be through personal relationships, through meaningful links with community or spiritual groups, or through a strong belief in the work you do. By redefining your core values on a regular basis, you will be able to organize your life to reflect these values, giving attention, priority, energy and time to the really important things in life rather than the trivia.

Closely linked to this is the fulfilment of personal spiritual needs, ensuring that we receive the nourishment and uplift we need. It is important to get our hearts and minds out of the hurly-burly of everyday life and into communion with our own spiritual nature and into connection with all that is around us. People suffer, often without even realizing it, from a deep spiritual malaise and a longing to touch the world of Spirit and 'the kingdom of heaven which is within'.

For many of us, everyday hassles can be transcended by going to places of great natural beauty or by getting in contact with nature. For others, exquisite music or the spontaneous excitement, joy and beauty of small children can lift them out of their normal, preoccupied state of mind. Some will tap into the essence of Divine love through human love and committed relationships, or through service to others. Creativity and self-expression is another major source of joy and spiritual well-being. And for yet others, spiritual connection and uplift will come through meditation or religious practice. While some will have a more immediate or gnostic sense of spirituality, enabling them to feel quite palpably the presence and love of the Holy Spirit, others will have their relationship with Spirit through their religious belief and the faith this generates.

Certainly, many who attend the Bristol Cancer Help Centre say it has been the recognition of their spiritual nature and the defining and prioritizing of their spiritual needs that have been responsible for their healing. The profound personal transformation they undergo as a result of opening up to the spiritual dimension and developing their own personal spirituality, can result in a wonderful new relationship to both life and death, and in many cases remarkable physical recovery as well.

If you are prepared to prioritize your peace of mind and spiritual well-being, your life will become simpler and enriched at the same time. This will enable you to feel you have 'come home' in a very profound and meaningful way. Most people who go through this process say they feel more and more alive and happier than ever before. And not only does their health improve greatly, but they also start to feel younger. This slowing down of the ageing process is very noticeable in people who are free and fulfilled spiritually. This very real phenomenon can be put down to the effects of a positive state of mind which creates measurable improvements in our immune system and tissue function.

The energy model of health

Looking at the body's underlying energy and vitality is another very important way of evaluating our state of health. In all traditional Eastern medicines, such as acupuncture, shiatsu, yoga and tai chi, the aim is to work with this underlying energy or 'life force', ensuring that all the different energies of the body are in balance and that overall energy levels are high. In acupuncture and tai chi this energy is called *chi*, in shiatsu *ki*, and in yoga, *prana*.

The Western equivalent of this energy is found in homeopathy, where it is referred to as the 'vital force'. It is actually quite easy, even without training in Oriental medicine, to sense whether a person's energy is basically in good shape. All of us make an 'energy diagnosis' when we look at our houseplants, judging whether they are full of life and vitality or not! People with good *chi* radiate health and are a pleasure to be around, whereas those who are low in energy or whose energy is out of balance often feel draining or uncomfortable to be with.

Nowadays, with high-tech photographic techniques, it is possible to see the body's energy field and begin to visualize for ourselves the subtle energy systems on which Oriental medicine is based. With new bio-energy measuring and treatment devices, such as the Russian Scenar or Kosmed device (see Appendix 1), the body's energy levels can be measured and treated at the same time.

Through modern physics, we now know categorically that all matter is fundamentally made of energy, and that living systems produce electrical fields. Our Oriental ancestors knew this thousands of years ago, and their ability to detect, assess and rebalance the subtle energies of the body says much about their sensitivity and consciousness. In the West, owing to a combination of poor diet, alcohol, cigarettes, stress, overwork, overstimulation and sedentary lifestyle, most of us are only experiencing about half our potential energy.

It is often helpful to visualize our energy, imagining we have a spectrum of energy levels from 0 to 100 per cent. We are usually born with very high energy levels, as all parents of small children will testify! But over time our lifestyles rob us of this vitality, leaving most of us only half way up the energy scale. At this level, people become susceptible to minor illness such as colds, flu and stomach upsets, and while they are generally able to work, many suffer from a lack of energy.

The energy model of health and illness

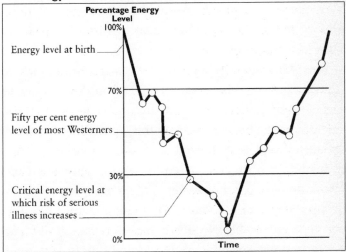

Overwork or adverse life events which cause upset, shock or disappointment, can take energy levels dangerously low, to a critical level of, say, 30 per cent. Below this point people are vulnerable to far more serious illnesses, and are likely to develop any health problem to which they are susceptible, whether it is asthma, schizophrenia or cancer. Another problem is that when energy levels drop, the mental state changes with it. When energy levels are low, self-esteem, confidence and motivation go out the window. People are also likely to become far more fearful and anxious, feel pain far more acutely, find it harder to sleep and feel that life is out of their control. In this situation they are on a slippery slope – from this point it is hard for them to take action to pull themselves out of the trough they have fallen into. In fact, at this point people often make things worse for themselves. When we feel things are getting out of control our response is often to try even harder, stressing and exhausting ourselves even more. As a result, people become even more depleted, and at the same time beat themselves up about their failure to 'deliver'.

A tell-tale sign of being in this low-energy state is when, even though we know what we need to do in order to increase our energy levels, we are unable to do it. Many people leading busy lives are in this state – they feel tired, exhausted and demoralized, and know they would feel heaps better if they exercised, relaxed or meditated but find it quite impossible to get to the gym or a meditation group. People in chronically low energy states like this are very vulnerable physically and psychologically, and are far more susceptible to developing cancer.

To reduce the risk of cancer, learning how to 'tune into' and assess our energy levels, listening very closely to what our bodies are telling us, is the first step. It is then vital to adjust our behaviour accordingly. The first and most obvious thing to do when working with our energy levels is to balance work with rest and recreation. But it is also important to learn how to raise our energy levels, through both therapeutic intervention and self-help techniques, which will be described later in this chapter.

As energy levels rise, the reverse situation occurs. When they reach, say, 70 per cent, psychological health starts to improve dramatically. People feel empowered – as if everything is going their way – and they often start to experience synchronicity or significant coincidences in life. In other words, as the lift in energy raises their consciousness, they experience meaningful insight into their own lives and have a far greater sense of connection to and support from life itself. People repeatedly say that once in this state, life and the things they want come towards them and they no longer have to struggle constantly to make things happen.

When energy levels drop below the 30 per cent level, it is usually necessary to receive therapeutic help to get back from this point. Therapies that will lift energy levels are: acupuncture, shiatsu, homeopathy and, especially, spiritual healing. Once energy levels are lifted out of the 'doldrums', it is possible to keep on building them up through self-help techniques such as relaxation, meditation, tai chi, yoga and exercise. All these therapies and self-help techniques will be described in detail later in this chapter.

Recovering vital energy

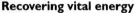

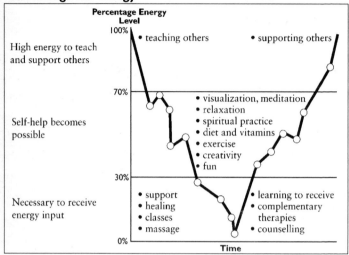

Caring for the body

The other major factor within the holistic health model is how we look after ourselves physically. Feeding ourselves properly and exercising regularly greatly affects our energy, vitality and state of mind. But it is not just about what food we eat, but also how we eat, where we shop, how we store food and how we cook it. It is very important to make changes to our diet that are sustainable, rather than flipping between periods of very healthy eating and binges on unhealthy food.

Combining forms of exercise that build stamina with those that increase suppleness, strength and harmonization of body, mind and spirit, is a good idea. The ideal combination is to take aerobic exercise, preferably outdoors, once or twice a week, and to do a weekly class in yoga, tai chi or chi gong as well, with a short daily practice of these disciplines at home.

CREATING YOUR OWN CANCER-PREVENTION PLAN

When reading the rest of this chapter it would be helpful to make notes so that you can start to form your own cancer-prevention plan. With each section, try to make a list of the changes you wish to make and how you are going to achieve them.

Healthy eating and cooking

A wholefood organic diet, which is very low in animal foods, fat, salt, sugar, processed foods, chemical additives, stimulants (such as tea and coffee) and alcohol, is what we all should aim towards. For most people, this will mean increasing dramatically their intake of vegetables, fruit, cereals and pulses while reducing their total calorie intake and changing everything 'white' in their diet to the 'brown' unprocessed equivalent. It will also mean drinking herbal teas, juices and mineral or filtered water, rather than tea and coffee.

Lynda McGilvray changed her diet completely after she was diagnosed with breast cancer at the age of thirty. Before the diagnosis in 1981, she had never really thought about what she ate and often relied on fast food, left-overs and ready-made meals. But after undergoing surgery and radiotherapy, she attended the Bristol Cancer Help Centre in a bid to find the support she needed. She was amazed at what she found there – everything made sense and it became a move that changed her life.

As well as learning meditation, relaxation and healing, Lynda adopted a vegan diet suggested by the Centre. In the first six weeks after leaving the Centre, she made dramatic changes to her diet, cutting out all meat, fish and dairy products and eating only vegetables and pulses. She also started taking a regime of vitamins and mineral supplements. To begin with it was hard for Lynda, whose children were young at the time. She found as soon as she had finished chopping vegetables for one meal, it was time to start on the next. But she persevered, and within two to three weeks felt cleansed, full of energy and in control. After six weeks, she went back to eating fish and chicken occasionally, and now eats fish twice a week. Over the last eighteen years, Lynda's diet has changed, but she is still very aware of what she should and should not eat. While there are still days when she eats less well, these are far outweighed by the good days.

Since the first diagnosis, Lynda has had two recurrences of breast cancer – one in 1988 and the second in 1996. But for the last four years there has been no sign of the disease and, at the age of forty-nine, she feels very good. Being diagnosed with cancer and the help Lynda received from the Bristol Cancer Help Centre and her local cancer support group, have completely changed her life. Now she has a much better outlook, and she feels she has gained a great deal of her new vitality and continued good health from healthy eating.

How to change the way you eat

Changing something as fundamental as the food you eat involves a great deal of commitment and support. It is very important to make changes in a way that is sustainable. Quite often, if changes are too radical or too quick, they are abandoned within weeks, especially if the new regime feels like a diet or a form of deprivation, leaving you with the desire to binge on 'naughty foods'. The other ingredients for success are getting the right sort of support to help you make the changes and acquiring the right information, recipes and new cooking skills.

Support

If you are going to start eating in a healthy way, it is vital to enlist the support of your partner, family, colleagues and friends. Also, if you are really serious about making this commitment to yourself, it is good to have 'witnesses'. The very process of telling people will make your intention seem more real. Obviously, it is better still if you can get the people you live with to make the changes too. This will avoid all sorts of conflicts about how you are going to shop, cook and prepare food – and the more nitty gritty issue of how the family budget is going to be spent! If you can't persuade your nearest and dearest to join in, then it is a good idea to find a 'buddy' or even a small gang of friends or colleagues who would like to make the changes with you.

If you can muster several people who want to change their diet, you could form your own 'healthy eating support group' and meet regularly for a few weeks to talk about how you are getting on and swap information and creative ideas. I have seen this work in an office environment, where a whole team decided to 'clean up their act' with regard to food. They supported each other very well by replacing biscuits and cakes with big bowls of fruit, sweetened drinks with mineral water and fruit juice, and tea and coffee with herbal teas. They also met weekly to discuss meal plans and their progress.

This group started with a healthy springcleaning 'detox' diet to lose weight. It revolved around eating only fruit, steamed vegetables, salads, soup and brown rice for six weeks. Thereafter, other new wholefoods were added to the healthy eating plan. The group members were delighted with the results, both in terms of weight loss and a marked improvement in energy levels and mental clarity. The feeling of solidarity among members was absolutely wonderful, and this also rubbed off on their work together.

If you recognize that you have a great emotional dependency on food, it may be necessary to get more than family or friends to support you, and going to a counsellor or doctor may be a good idea. Once you start to eat less heavy foods, which are sedating, you may well uncover anxieties and feelings that have been lurking under the surface for years. If this occurs, it is unlikely that you will be able to change your eating patterns successfully until you get therapeutic help. Counselling can help people to offload their emotions and change long term the way they deal with their feelings. Agencies through which you can find a counsellor are listed in Appendix 1.

Information

Getting information about how to cook healthy food has never been easier. Healthy eating is talked and written about frequently these days and there are many extremely good cookery and nutrition books available that give step-by-step advice on what to do (see Appendix 1). Before you start your new diet you will need the following:

- dietary advice explaining what to eat and what not to eat.

- a clear idea of what healthy foods are available and what you should buy.

- a meal plan to take you through the first few weeks.

- nutritional information to ensure what you are eating is balanced and healthy.

- a good set of recipes.

- professional advice if you have special dietary needs as a result of illness or disabilities.

- information on how to store and cook foods to gain maximum nutritional value.

This information will be explained step by step in the following pages. But if this all seems too much, the whole operation can be made far simpler by going to a nutritional therapist for one-to-one help in successfully making the change-over. A nutritional therapist is not the same as a dietician. Most dieticians are trained in the standard Western diet and how to adjust this for certain illnesses or conditions. In general, they will happily recommend a diet based on meat, dairy foods and refined carbohydrates. Nutritional therapists, on the other hand, look at the role of food itself – as a cause and treatment of illness – and tend to advocate a wholefood, healthy diet. Planning changes to your diet with a professional can make all the difference to your chance of success and is highly recommended. (See Appendix 1 for information on finding a nutritional therapist.)

Dietary guidelines
Key advice for a healthy diet:

- Eat fruit and/or vegetables at every single meal. Include a high proportion of raw fruit and vegetables every day, either on their own or in salads or home-made vegetable juices, which are an excellent source of nutrition. (Commercially available fruit and vegetable juices have to be pasteurized by law. Part of this process involves heating the juice which destroys health-giving plant enzymes, so the homemade variety is much better.) For making juices at home you will read a basic juice extractor (costing around £50) or a better, more expensive juice press such as the Champion Juicer.

- Get as much variety in your diet as possible and try different pulses, fruits and vegetables. This will ensure you get the full spectrum of minerals and vitamins and the vital plant phytochemicals necessary to prevent cancer.

- Replace refined and processed foods with the wholefood, unprocessed equivalent. This means replacing white bread with brown bread; white rice with brown rice; white pasta with brown pasta; ordinary cheese biscuits with oatcakes: sugary cakes with fruit cakes; normal breakfast cereal with muesli or porridge; sweets and chocolate with nuts, dried fruits or ordinary fruit; and sweetened drinks with mineral water, fruit or vegetable juice (preferably homemade).

- Replace red meat and farmed chicken and fish with vegetable protein from beans, lentils, peas and quinoa, with occasional use of organic deep-sea fish, wild salmon or trout, free-range organic chicken or game, free-range organic eggs – and very occasionally use of organic red meat.

- Replace most animal fats with vegetarian equivalents. The exception to this rule are the fish oils which contain essential omega-3 fatty acids. They are found in oily fish such as mackerel, herrings or salmon (organic), or you can take fish oil tablets. Replace whole milk with skimmed milk or, better still, with vegetable drinks such as soya, oat or rice milk. You could try cutting milk from the diet altogether by drinking weak black tea and using fruit juices on muesli for breakfast. Porridge can be eaten without milk, flavoured with fruit concentrates or date or maple syrup.

- Replace cheese with vegetable pâtés, such as olive, aubergine, avocado (guacamole) and mushroom. It is also better to use a fish pâté than cheese. But check pâtés or pastes are not full of 'hidden' cream cheese.

- Replace animal cooking fat with vegetable oils –

preferably cold-pressed olive oil or groundnut oil. Use speciality oils such as sesame oil and walnut oil for flavouring salad dressings.

- Replace cream with soya cream and ice cream with soya ice cream.

- Replace normal yoghurts with soya desserts and yoghurts such as Provamel.

- Replace butter with vegetable equivalents such as olive oil-based spreads. Many margarines are unhealthy because they are highly processed and contain hydrogenated and trans-fatty acids. These are produced by excessive heating of the fats in the production process. Margarines which do not contain hydrogenated fatty acids include Vitaquel and Granose, which can be used as an alternative to olive oil-based spreads.

Faced with this advice, most people panic that they will not get sufficient protein and calcium for healthy growth and bones. At this point, I usually remind people that huge creatures like elephants and cows are vegetarian and they have no problem whatsoever maintaining their huge bone structure and health.

In reality, most people in developed countries eat far too much protein every day. It is estimated that we actually need only 40 grams (just over 1 ounce) of protein a day to replace the wear and tear on our joints and muscles. All the basic vitamins and minerals we need are available from a varied vegan diet. Over the years, the meat and milk marketing boards have done a very good job at convincing us that good health depends entirely on our intake of dairy food, meat and eggs. Just try to hold clearly in your mind the fact that most degenerative health problems in the West are due to over-eating and, in particular, to the excessive consumption of animal fats and meat.

Buying healthy food

If wholefood is new to you, the best thing to do is go to a good health food shop and see exactly what is on offer. You will be amazed by the huge selection of raw ingredients on display, as well as pre-prepared vegan and vegetarian meals. Of course, many of these healthy foods, such as pulses, seeds, nuts, dried fruits and wholefood cereals, are available in supermarkets too. But since most supermarkets stock only a small proportion of healthy food, it is worth going to a speciality wholefood shop first, to see the full range and to familiarize yourself with what is available. Supermarkets are now taking on board the healthy-eating message and more and more are launching healthy food ranges as well as selling organic fruit and vegetables. So once you know what you are looking for, it may well be possible to return to your normal supermarket.

Recipe books

Health food shops will often have a book section too, where you can pick from a range of both European and Oriental vegetarian options. Quite often, Indian or Middle Eastern vegetarian cookery is a good option for those who are used to a very elaborate diet and tend to find vegetarian food a bit boring. The main problem with basic vegetarian meals is that they can at first seem bland in comparison with the intensity of flavours and the variation of textures involved in traditional cooking. However, the exotic recipes and the diversity of Oriental cookery methods and ingredients overcome this problem very well. Any good high street bookshop will have a vegetarian section in the cookery department, and often health food shops have a particularly good book selection. (See Appendix 1 for cookbook suggestions.)

Wholefood shopping

On your first trip to the wholefood shop or good supermarket, a basic shopping list would include:

- brown rice, pasta and flour

- beans

- lentils

- sugar-free high-quality muesli and porridge oats

- good-quality organic wholemeal bread

- nuts, seeds and dried fruit

- vegetable pâté or hummus

- herbal tea

- mineral water

- wholefood biscuits and cake

- soya, oat or rice milk

- soya yoghurt or dessert

- olive oil spread, or Granose or Vitaquel margarine

- olive oil

- tamari or soy sauce for flavouring foods (as an alternative to salt)

In addition to these basics, building up a selection of herbs, spices and specialist ingredients is a good idea to help flavour vegetarian food in interesting ways. Useful ingredients are garlic, ginger, balsamic vinegar, chilli sauce and tomato purée, as well as interesting options like chestnut purée and coconut cream. It is also possible to buy soya mayonnaise, which is not nearly so high in fat as ordinary mayonnaise. Excellent green and red curry pastes from Thailand are available, as are delightful favourings such as lemongrass, star anise and Chinese five spice, along with the fresh herbs coriander, rosemary, thyme and bay. Soya desserts mixed with fresh fruit can be made far more interesting by marinating the soya with vanilla pods and star anise, together with a little honey or maple syrup. Tomatoes served with freshly chopped basil, olive oil and balsamic vinegar, salt and pepper are an absolute delight.

Fruit concentrates, such as apple and strawberry, can be used very effectively to flavour sauces, desserts and cakes, as can maple and date syrups. Soaking dried fruits with herbs is another delicious option. For example, soaking Hunza apricots with bay leaves and cardamoms prior to cooking transforms this dish into a completely magical, gourmet experience. If you try this idea, soak the apricots overnight with the bay and cardamoms, then bring them to the boil and simmer for five to ten minutes. Leave to steep for a further twenty-four hours before serving to thicken and enrich the juice. Served with soya cream, this dish is indeed proof that healthy food can be just as rich and delicious as more conventional food – and in no way equals deprivation!

An introductory meal plan

The better the structure of a new diet, the more successful it is likely to be. A meal plan for one week is a good idea to begin with, and it can either be repeated or changed at the beginning of each new week.

Breakfast should include some of the following:

- fresh fruit, fresh fruit salad, or a dried fruit compote (soaked overnight)

- healthy cereal such as muesli or porridge (which can be made from many other cereals besides oats)

- brown toast with high-quality, low-sugar fruit spreads or honey

- boiled eggs (occasionally)

- fruit juice or herbal teas (if you are going to drink tea or coffee, try to do this only once or twice a day and drink herbal teas or mineral water the rest of the time; it is better for your teeth (and your children's teeth) to drink fruit juice at meal times only)

Decide which is going to be your main meal – lunch or dinner – and swap the following meals around accordingly.

A light lunch could include a choice of:

- vegetable or fish soup

- fresh salad, bean salad or rice salad

- a wholefood vegetarian pasty, pie, samosa or falafels

- wholewheat bread or toast with vegetable pâté, tomatoes and rocket

- fresh fruit, fruit salad or stewed fruit

For dinner you could choose from:

- pasta with tomato or mushroom sauce, vegetarian bolognaise or pesto

- vegetable curries and dahl with rice

- lentil shepherd's pie with vegetables

- stir-fried vegetables with rice

- vegetable stews, baked or stuffed vegetables

- nut roast

- wholefood fruit desserts, pies, crumbles and bakes

All of the above should be accompanied by a fresh salad and/or steamed vegetables. It is also fine to include organic fish, game or meat on an occasional basis.

Nutritional information

A healthy diet includes a good balance of:

- protein

- carbohydrates (starch and sugar)

- essential fatty acids

- fruit and vegetables

Vegetarian protein comes from beans, peas, lentils, nuts, seeds and the delicious cereal quinoa (which contains all twenty-one amino acids we need). *Carbohydrates* are available from bread, pasta, potatoes and other root vegetables. *Essential fatty acids* are obtained from nuts, seeds, vegetables and fish oils. With all these foods, make sure you have as much variety as possible. All these healthy wholefoods have a different balance of vitamins and minerals, and for optimum health it is best to vary your intake and experiment with new pulses, fruits and vegetables. Jane Sen, of the Bristol Cancer Help Centre, says that an easy way to be sure you are getting the full range of nutrients is to mix vegetables and foods of different colours in one meal. If you are worried about getting the right nutritional balance, especially for children or the elderly, again the advice is to invest in some time with a nutritional therapist or buy a good wholefood nutrition text book (see Appendix 1). The most important thing to remember is that you *can* get all the nutrients you need from a vegetarian diet.

Another concern people have about changing to a wholefood diet is that they will lose too much weight.

Usually, when people make the change they lose some weight initially as refined sugars and animal fats are dropped from the diet. For example, one chocolate and toffee bar can contain the same amount of sugar as about fifteen apples! However, people on a wholefood diet are satisfied long before eating this many apples, and therefore consume far less sugar whilst getting all the healthy vitamins, minerals, phytochemicals and fibre they need. After a while, weight normally reaches a new healthy equilibrium. If it continues to fall, you are probably concentrating too much on fruit and vegetables and not getting enough carbohydrate and fat. In this case, it may be helpful to seek the advice of a nutritional therapist to find out where you are going wrong.

A great added bonus of changing to a healthy cancer-prevention diet is that other illnesses you may have will start to clear up. The most common improvements are in asthma, eczema, arthritis, migraine and gut complaints. Many of these illnesses are caused by allergies to animal foods, or by lack of the right mineral, vitamin and plant phytochemicals – problems which are rectified with a healthy, vegetable-based diet. People also have far less mucus, and the throat, ears and sinuses feel much clearer. This means fewer infections too. Other benefits include an increase in energy levels, clarity of mind, and healthy skin. In fact, most people who make these changes ask themselves why on earth it took them so long to do so, because they feel so much lighter, clearer and so very much more alive.

Specific anti-cancer foods

All vegetables, nuts, seeds and pulses contain some of the vital cancer-preventing phytochemicals, and so eating the widest range possible of these foods is essential. However, some foods have particularly high levels of these protective plant chemicals and you should make sure your cancer-prevention diet is high in these ingredients. This area has been brilliantly researched by nutritionist Suzannah Olivier, who has compiled the following list of foods which help to prevent cancer. The full list of the phytochemicals they contain is in Appendix 2. For a full explanation of the scientifically researched properties of individual phytochemicals, I thoroughly recommend Suzannah Olivier's book *The Breast Cancer Prevention and Recovery Diet* (see Appendix 1).

Anti-cancer foods: alfalfa; onions; spring onions; garlic; leeks; chives; almonds; apples; broccoli; cabbage; Brussels sprouts; kale; bok choy; kohl rabi; arugula; horse radish; radish; swede; turnip; sprouted broccoli and cauliflower seeds; burdock root; citrus foods; flax oil; ginger; grapes; licorice; linseeds; the Oriental mushrooms maitake, reishei and shiitake; nettles; almonds; walnuts; black walnuts; pecans; sunflower seeds; sesame seeds; olive oil; apricots; cantaloupe melons; carrots; yellow and red peppers; beetroot; squash; sweet potatoes; red and black berries; parsley; pineapple; potatoes; pulses and beans; brown rice; the seaweeds kombu, kelp, nori, arame, laver bread, dulse and wakame; soy products; black tea; green tea; tomatoes; turmeric.

Learning new culinary skills

There is no way around the fact that changing to a whole-food, vegetarian diet will involve acquiring new skills. You may be fortunate enough to have access to a whole-food cookery class through a local college of further education or cookery school. Local nutritional therapists may also teach or know about courses on wholefood cookery, as might the people who run local health food shops, restaurants or natural health clinics. Again, a good whole-food recipe book will offer many ideas and vital guidance on how to master these basic skills. But the simplest way is to find somebody who already eats healthily who can teach you the first steps. These will include learning to:

- cook brown rice, pulses, grains and cereals successfully.

- stir-fry and bake vegetables.

- make a good variety of salads which include raw vegetables, seeds, nuts, fruits and cooked pulses as well as the usual salad ingredients.

- make vegetable soups and juices.

- make wholefood cakes, biscuits and desserts.

- make basic sauces and dressings with healthy ingredients.

Sustainability

In order to sustain the changes you make, the golden rule is to start adding healthy foods to your diet before you take other things out. For example, try first to get into the habit of eating fruit and vegetables with every single meal.

The next step is to replace all processed 'white' foods with the brown equivalent. Because these foods are so much more sustaining than their 'white' counterparts, you will soon start to find that your blood sugar level is less inclined to dip, which is what makes you want to reach for sugary snacks and drinks. The desire to eat sweets and savoury snacks between meals will gradually reduce. Once this starts to happen, your appetite will level out and it will then be possible to drop richer and heavier foods such as meats and animal fats. In a short time you will feel so much better that you will wonder how you survived so long eating in such an unhealthy way.

Healthy cooking
Barbecuing, smoking and microwaving foods (especially meat and meat fats) are the cooking methods to avoid. It is also best to avoid overheating fat when frying and, in particular, to avoid the repeated use of oils for deep frying. Over-heated oils and smoke from barbecues and food-smoking processes produce dangerous free radicals in food, which can be carcinogenic. It is therefore advisable to keep clear of barbecued, smoked and char-grilled meats and fish and to restrict frying to a minimum. When you do fry food, always use new oil and do not heat it until it smokes. This is a sure sign that the fat is beginning to superheat and break down into free radicals.

The best cooking methods are:

- steaming
- stir-frying
- stewing

- roasting

- baking

With steaming and stir-frying, foods can be cooked quickly and lightly, thereby retaining much of their natural texture and nutrients. Baking, roasting and stewing are gentler ways of cooking than frying or grilling and allow flavours to melt into one another at lower temperatures. Believe it or not, it is actually possible to 'fry' foods in a little water. Heat a small amount of water in a frying pan and cook the food exactly as if you were frying it. You can then add good-quality cold-pressed oils (like olive, sesame or walnut) at the end of cooking for flavour and nutritional value. By cooking in this way, you will appreciate the flavours of the oil far more than when it is overheated and broken down in frying.

When stir-frying use a minimum amount of oil – just enough to stop vegetables or other foods sticking to the wok or frying pan. Steaming is the healthiest cooking method because foods that are steamed retain maximum flavour and texture (in contrast to those that are boiled which leak vital nutrients (particularly minerals) and flavours into the cooking water). With steaming, there is only a slight leakage of nutrients into the steaming water. Whether steaming or boiling food, it is a good idea to use the cooking water in other recipes, such as soups, stews and sauces.

When you change to healthy eating, one of the best things to master is the making of really good and varied salads. In Britain, people are brought up with the idea that a salad comprises lettuce, tomato and cucumber. But in reality the range of possibilities is enormous. What works particularly well is grated raw vegetables mixed with conventional salad foods, sprouted seeds and pulses. Grated carrots and beetroot, finely chopped courgettes or broccoli, mixed with sprouts, watercress, rocket and tomatoes, for example, make a stunning salad. Pre-cooked beans are another good ingredient. Red kidney beans with chopped tomatoes, parsley, a little chopped onion and a good garlic dressing make a very nutritious and delicious meal.

Try also making salads with grains such as rice, quinoa, bulgar wheat and cous cous, and experiment with different dressings. Most of us get locked into using oil and vinegar, but wonderful dressings can be made with other ingredients. For example, try puréed, skinned fresh tomatoes and basil with a little lime, lemon or vinegar, salt and pepper.

Another good skill to acquire is the ability to sprout seeds and pulses. This can be done in jam jars or other glass containers. The secret is first to soak the seeds or pulses in double their volume of water for the first day, drain and rinse them on the second day, leaving them damp in the jar to germinate. Rinse them again each day until the sprouts are ready to eat. The best seeds and beans to sprout are alfalfa, mung, aduki and chick peas.

Useful equipment
To make wholefood cooking easier, it is worth investing in a good food processor because you will be preparing more vegetables and salads. This will chop and grate

vegetables extremely quickly. Also, invest in a juice extractor or press so that you can use pure vegetable and fruit
juices, both for drinks and to make delicious sauces and
soups. It is also a good idea to get a vegetable steamer.
The most useful one is a little collapsible steamer which
fits inside an ordinary pan. It is circular with petals that
open like a flower so it fits different sizes of pans, and is
available from all good cookware shops. If you have a
large family and are likely to be doing a lot of steaming,
you could invest in a more elaborate, multi-level steamer
in which you can cook three types of vegetables simultaneously. A hand blender and chopping set can also be
invaluable for making soups or vegetable purées in the
pan they've been cooked in, vinaigrettes and for chopping herbs for sauces. If you can, get an electric coffee
grinder too, but keep it solely for grinding nuts, seeds
and spices such as nutmeg. As mentioned earlier you
should also buy a juice extractor or press if affordable.

For stir-frying it is worth investing in a Chinese wok.
This is what the Chinese use for most of their cookery. It
looks a bit like a frying pan but has a gentle curved shape
and a long wooden handle. It is designed in this way so
that it is easier to keep tossing the contents of the wok
gently during cooking, which ensures everything in the
pan gets cooked quickly and evenly without burning or
over-cooking. A good set of knives is helpful for peeling
and chopping vegetables, and another handy tool is a
small mandolin-style vegetable peeler (which does the job
much quicker than a standard peeler). It is also good to
have a dedicated electric coffee grinder or a pestle and
mortar to grind seeds, nuts and spices.

Vitamin, mineral and
herbal supplements

The main vitamins, minerals and plant-food supplements which are protective against cancer are:

- the antioxidant vitamins C, E and betacarotene (the safe form of vitamin A)

- the minerals zinc and selenium (involved in the enzymes which are used in antioxidant processes)

- naturally occurring antioxidants and plant phyto-chemicals (condensed and sold as plant-food supplement)

- vitamin D (protects the bowel against cancer)

- low-dose aspirin (has also been shown to protect against bowel cancer)

Some people say it is not necessary to take vitamin and mineral supplements to prevent cancer if you are eating a healthy diet. But I disagree, because most of us are exposed to high levels of stress and chemical toxicity in the environment. I believe it is a good idea to take basic vitamin and mineral supplements to boost the immune system and provide background antioxidant support to our tissues. However, smokers should not take beta-carotene. Recent research has shown that while people with high blood levels of betacarotene are protected against cancer, smokers who rapidly increase their levels of betacarotene are more likely to develop lung cancer.

The reason for this is not yet understood. My message to smokers is: first, give up smoking (take vitamins and minerals during this process, as suggested on page 125), then add in betacarotene when the smoke is well and truly out of your system, after around three months. Recent controversy about vitamin C has been misleading. Overall there is still overwhelming evidence in favour of the use of vitamin C to prevent cancer. The suggestion that vitamin C can actually cause DNA damage is not supported by the scientists who did the trials themselves! These scientists say that oxidative change seen in DNA with vitamin C, which could be construed as DNA damage, is the first of two steps in an overall DNA repair process triggered by vitamin C.

Suggested supplements and dosages (iu = international units) for cancer prevention and optimum health are:

- vitamin C (500 mg three times a day)

- betacarotene (15 mg a day), but not recommended for smokers

- vitamin E (400 iu a day). If you are taking anticoagulant drugs let your GP know you are also planning to take vitamin E because it has a slightly anticoagulant effect

- selenium (200 iu a day)

- vitamin B complex (50 mg once a day)

- multivitamin tablets (one a day) which contain some

vitamin D and zinc as well as the full spectrum of other
minerals and vitamins needed to maintain health

By having at least one glass of freshly prepared vegetable
juice every day, you will ensure these supplements are
used optimally by the body. It will allow all the naturally
occurring co-factors and enzymes from the vegetables to
support the body's use of extra vitamins and minerals.

In good health food shops, you will also find products
which have been designed with cancer prevention in
mind. These contain a good range of the phytochemicals,
vitamins and minerals that are known to be helpful,
usually in the form of either powders or liquids to be
taken daily. There is no doubt that these products will
make you feel fantastic, as well as convey excellent protection. Of particular value are plant supplements which
contain catechins. These are the elements of green tea
which are so protective. Also available now, in tablet form,
is the active anti-cancer ingredient from the brassica
family. It is called indole-3-carbinol and the daily protective dose is 300 mg. Two other food concentrates which
significantly boost immune function and protect against
cancer are MGN 3 (a mushroom extract) and IP6 (a deriv-
ative of vitamin B). Among other effects, they both significantly raise levels of the all-important immune 'natural
killer cells' which are known to destroy cancer cells.

If your family history puts you at greater risk of bowel
cancer, it is wise to take a vitamin D supplement and 300 mg
of enteric coated aspirin daily. This type of aspirin is
designed to be broken down once it has gone through the
stomach, helping to prevent stomach ulcers developing.

Taking extra calcium and folic acid is also believed to reduce colon cancer risk. Studies have shown that legumes and beans protect against uterine cancer and, astonishingly, that strawberries and raspberries protect against cancer of the cervix!

Protection against cancer of the prostate is achieved by taking vitamin E. Some scientists recommend 50 mg per day, which is around 75 iu. Others recommend as much as 800 iu. I recommend a level of 400 iu for men and women as an important element of overall cancer prevention.

Anti-cancer herbs include essiac (an American Indian medicine) and carctol (an Indian Ayurvedic medicine). These can be taken at maintenance dose levels as part of a cancer-prevention plan. Another intriguing proposition is to make and drink kombuchu, a sour drink which is believed to have anti-cancer properties. Like ginger beer, it is generated from a 'plant' or culture which grows and requires splitting regularly.

Exercise

Exercise is a vital element of cancer prevention because it cleans out the tissues of the body. When we exercise, blood flow increases to all parts of the body, bringing oxygen, nutrients and white blood cells to the tissues. This in turn promotes the flow of blood in both the veins and lymph glands away from the tissues, taking toxins to the kidneys, liver, skin and lungs for excretion. As previously mentioned, in traditional Oriental medicine, disease is believed to develop in areas of 'stagnation' within the body. In acupuncture or shiatsu, this is seen as stagnation of energy, or *chi*. But the concept of stagnation can also be applied to a physical process – when for example, tissues and joints literally silt up with toxins from our diet and the breakdown products of alcohol, drugs and cigarettes. Fat, calcium, heavy metals and organic chemical residues from environmental pollution are deposited directly in the tissues, as are the breakdown products of radiation. So it is easy to see how tissues become more and more toxic, creating the ideal environment for cancer to develop. It is not surprising therefore that exercise lowers cancer rates. Certainly, women who exercise are 10 to 20 per cent less likely to develop breast cancer than those who do not. This shows that exercise represents a very significant contribution to overall protection against cancer.

But which sort of exercise is best? In the holistic approach to health, Oriental exercises such as yoga, tai chi and chi gong are favoured. This is because they are very intelligently designed to involve every single tissue, joint and organ, bringing blood and vital energy to all parts of the body. In addition, they incorporate elements of relaxation, deep breathing and meditation, which produce strong benefits through the mind–body connection. They can also generate a very harmonious and respectful attitude to life, laying good foundations for the development of a spiritual practice.

Yoga is a multi-level process in which learning the postures (or asanas) is only one of the seven pathways towards complete health, happiness, 'right living' and, ultimately, spiritual enlightenment. Of course, it is up to each individual how far he or she wishes to take the study of yoga. But even at the most basic level of attending a weekly class which combines a mixture of postures with some relaxation, meditation and breathing exercises (*pranayama*), the benefits to health and well-being are phenomenal. It is best to find a teacher through the British Wheel of Yoga. He or she will have had an excellent training and have extremely high teaching standards (see Appendix 1).

Tai chi is the exercise you may have seen in films practised by the Chinese early in the morning or in the evening in a park. Again, the benefits of tai chi go very deep, and its practice is highly recommended as a form of cancer prevention. Chi gong comes from the same roots as tai chi but tends to be used when people are already ill. Chi gong literally means 'energy work' and the practice is usually tailored to the needs of individuals to help them rebalance and strengthen themselves in mind, body and spirit in order to overcome a particular health problem. Certainly, in the West, because most of us have allowed our physical health to degenerate, chi gong is just as beneficial as yoga and tai chi, and is particularly relevant if you already have health problems. (See Appendix 1 for tai chi and chi gong contacts.)

Because a relaxed body and calm mind are so essential in cancer prevention, these Oriental forms of exercise are strongly recommended. However, there is still a very important role for good old-fashioned aerobic exercise such as running, swimming and other sports. It is particularly good if you can take some of your aerobic exercise in the fresh air. The ideal would be go to a weekly class of yoga, tai chi or chi gong, and try to do at least fifteen to twenty minutes a day of stretching or exercising in one of these disciplines at home. This could be complemented by one or two sessions of aerobic exercise a week, one of which is outdoors.

In addition, try to walk whenever you can rather than taking the car, and make sure you do some form of stretching every day. If you cannot do yoga, tai chi or chi gong techniques, carry out your own stretch routine. Stretch your arms up above your head to extend your spine, do side bends to stretch your waist, and try to incorporate a spinal twist too. As well as helping to prevent cancer, this will make a huge difference to your posture, vitality and well-being, not to mention your looks. If you are not keen to try Oriental exercise, then the next best thing is to swim regularly. Swimming also exercises every single part of the body and can be a relaxing form of exercise.

If you have difficulties with your mobility and all this seems out of your reach, think again – it is possible to do many yoga stretches while sitting in a chair or even in bed. Tapes are available to help you adapt yoga to your own physical state (see Appendix 1). There are also hydrotherapy exercise classes in most good swimming pools for those who are limited physically. In fact, if your mobility is limited, then it is even more important to try to get involved in some form of physical exercise. If this is not possible, you could perhaps have a weekly massage. A good masseur can help shift toxins out of the body by a massage technique called lymph drainage (see Appendix 1).

Dealing with stress, anxiety and overwork

Stress, anxiety and overwork are usually connected to each other in a horrible, vicious cycle. If you are anxious about money, work performance or making a good impression on others, in order to get promotion or bonuses, affection or sex, you are likely to push yourself harder and harder at work, at home or in social situations. The resulting stress is exacerbated further if you are the sort of person who takes on more and more without thinking through the cost in terms of finance, time, energy and personal compromise. If you are also a perfectionist or workaholic and have high integrity but poor self-esteem, the demands you make on yourself can become ridiculous.

Stress in the early stages is a form of excitement or a healthy response to a challenge or threat. In fact, in the early stages, stress can greatly improve performance. A healthy stress level can bring out the best in people, helping them to break through the inertia or laziness that makes them underachieve. However, the greater the anxiety, the pressure and the fear of failure, the higher stress levels soar, to the point where people go beyond optimum performance. When this happens, they work harder and harder but achieve less and less. At this point there is serious risk of 'burn out'. Individuals will start displaying the tell-tale signs, such as inappropriate emotional reactions, bad decisions and failure to meet deadlines, and they will feel an ever-increasing sense of panic, despair and helplessness as their situation gets further and further out of control. This stage is sometimes accompanied by physical exhaustion, which actually prevents people from working harder. But if their stamina is good, individuals will often respond to these feelings by trying to drive themselves even harder, until they are literally forced to stop by a mental breakdown or physical illness.

In Western society, high stress and anxiety levels are reaching epidemic proportions. A combination of factors – the cost of living; the complexity of the roles, demands and expectations we all face, with many people tending to drive themselves very hard – is putting our health and well-being at very grave risk. And this is before we take into account the personal tragedy of discovering that we have managed to squeeze all the joy, fun, creativity and, often, love out of life.

Various studies have shown that stress puts people at greater risk of cardiovascular disease, high blood pressure, heart attacks and strokes. But what has not been so clearly emphasized is the effect that this kind of stress has on the immune system, predisposing us to cancer and infection at one extreme and allergic and autoimmune diseases at the other.

If you recognize you are in a spiralling cycle of stress, you must take action immediately. This applies as much to people who are in formal work as to those who are not. Many people who are out of work or who are at home looking after small children, get just as stressed as people with high-powered jobs and important positions. In fact, it has been shown that where stress is linked to power, the negative effects on health are not as great as when it is associated with powerlessness. Caring for sick relatives, elderly parents or small children, with all the juggling of tasks and priorities that this involves, combined with the personal sacrifices, frustration and lack of personal space and time to achieve your own goals, can also make people severely stressed. Indeed, any situation where there are deep and complex conflicting emotions can trigger stress, in the same way that overactivity can.

Stress has two major components. One is so-called 'external stress', which comes from your environment and your relationship to it. This covers everything from the stress of heavy work deadlines, trying to drive across a busy city at rush hour, living or working in a hostile environment, getting married or divorced, losing a loved one, or going on holiday, to the need to raise enough money to pay the mortgage and bills each month.

The second component is 'internal stress'. This is stress that arises as a result of your relationship with yourself. Most people are fairly conscious of the first form of stress, but are largely unconscious of the ways they stress themselves. Because internal stress tends to mirror our early life experiences and upbringing, our relationship with ourselves often reflects the type of relationship we had with key adults in our childhood. For example, if you had a harsh, critical, judgmental parent, then the chances are you will have adopted these qualities in your own personality and in your relationship with yourself. If so, you will be very likely to criticize yourself mercilessly, and push yourself harder and harder to achieve the kinds of results that this harsh parent would have found acceptable.

Perhaps even more common are people who have not

received the love and affection they needed. They will stress themselves interminably by trying to win love and approval from others, putting themselves through all kinds of hoops in order to do this. So it is more often than not our relationship with ourselves and our past history that determines the level of external stress we put ourselves through. Where we live, how we work, and the demands we make on ourselves and others will frequently come from our underlying sense of 'who we are' and 'what we should be doing' with our lives. For example, if you were brought up in affluent surroundings, had a public school education and enjoyed foreign holidays and designer clothes, you are very likely to put immense pressure on yourself to keep this type of lifestyle going. To this extent, many of us are 'victims' of a large number of relatively unconscious forces which push us into lifestyles that make us miserable. The whole question of our relationship with ourselves, and how to change this, will be addressed in Chapter 5. Meanwhile, the remainder of this chapter focuses on how to become aware of your stress levels and make practical changes to bring them under control.

Looking for signs of stress
Most of us know if we are stressed. We feel anxious, irritable, miserable and pressured. Physical signs of stress include a rapid, racing heartbeat, palpitations (where the heart misses a beat or jumps about irregularly), shallow breathing, indigestion, diarrhoea or constipation (sometimes accompanied by piles). As stress levels become severe, people become less effective in everything they

do. This may be very difficult to own up to, but it is better if you can spot this before it is pointed out to you by others – especially at work.

At this point people often say, 'I feel like I am running as fast as I can but I just can't keep up – in fact I feel like I'm going backwards.' This can be followed by feelings of complete despair, because they are already working as fast as they can and are facing collapse. With severe stress like this, it becomes impossible to distinguish between key tasks and trivia. People are often only able to deal with the tip of the iceberg – coping with what is immediately in front of them, answering phone calls and letters – and failing to do any strategic thinking or planning to make sure life will run smoothly and efficiently.

Another alarming symptom of severe stress is 'thought block', when mid-sentence you can't remember what it was you were talking about. Sometimes, when stress levels are really high, this can lead to full-blown panic attacks. Then ordinary anxiety spirals into terror and people become so paralysed by fear that it is impossible to think clearly. At this point, medical help is often required.

If you have any of these symptoms or are driving colleagues or family members into stress through your behaviour, it is extremely important to stop now and address these issues in order to help prevent cancer and other serious illnesses.

Reducing stress levels
The practical way of dealing with stress has two fundamental approaches. The first is to tackle the symptoms of

stress through relaxation, exercise and meditation. Learning how to meditate or relax will be described fully later in this chapter, and healthy exercise has been covered on pages 211–14. The second approach is to re-organize your day, at home or work, to remove any unnecessary sources of stress, prioritizing those activities which are absolutely necessary.

Nine times out of ten, reducing stress levels will mean simplifying your life, and this means having to let things go. People who are stressed almost always have needs, commitments and expectations that are beyond their ability to 'deliver' – at work or financially or emotionally. Getting life so out of balance is nearly always a sign of displaced emotional need, combined with a sense that everything will be all right if only something can be achieved, sorted out or bought.

When stress has become severe, most people need a break of two to four weeks with support and therapeutic help in order to allow the body to rebalance itself. In this situation, it is wise to start a programme of relaxation, counselling, and physical therapies such as massage, aromatherapy, reflexology and spiritual healing in order to help equilibrium become re-established. Counselling is usually necessary because people, when they become stressed, often tend to suppress emotion – or indeed it may be that emotion has caused the stress in the first place. If the above options are not available, it is good to try to let yourself sleep and rest as deeply as possible. Spiritual healing is often available on a donation basis, and can be an invaluable source of support at these times. If you cannot get to a healer, you could try absent healing through the National Federation of Spiritual Healers (see Appendix 1).

In the further reaches of stress and burn out, it is usually not possible to think clearly enough to re-organize your priorities and simplify your life. It is therefore wise not to even try until your stress levels have fallen after an initial phase of rest and therapeutic input. Part of the problem of stress is that people can no longer 'see the wood for the trees', which makes it very difficult to prioritize.

Once your stress levels have come down again, it is a good idea to sit down with either your family or work team and discuss the problem. Without a doubt, if you are feeling stressed, those around you will be stressed too. By taking a grip on the situation, you will be doing everybody in your immediate circle a favour. At first this might make you feel very vulnerable. But if you can get the support of your family or colleagues this will ultimately be a very helpful and bonding process. Explain to everyone that you are making a radical re-appraisal of the way you live your life. If you can get them on-side before you start, you will meet far less resistance and may even experience some solidarity.

At work, you may have to seek the help of an external consultant to manage organizational stress or see where you are losing efficiency and building stress into your system. You may also need to work with a mentor to learn new, more effective ways of running your working life. In your personal life, a stress or debt counsellor may be needed to help you sort out your problems, priorities and goals.

You need to be aware that this simplifying or letting-go process will inevitably involve some disappointment, as things you have been struggling to achieve are given up. However, what you may discover longer term is that paradoxically, as you do less you start to achieve more. This can clearly be seen when you start to meditate. When a proper meditation routine is established, life becomes much easier and, as stated before, things you have planned or visualized start coming to you and you no longer have to struggle to make them happen all the time. It is absolutely remarkable how, when you start to 'get yourself out of the way', the underlying process of life can start to support you.

Overcoming severe stress
The golden rules for bringing severe stress under control are:

1   Take a good two- to six-week break from all normal activity. In addition, work out a stress-busting programme of relaxation, massage and exercise to lessen the grip of stress on the body, and counselling to unburden yourself emotionally. Do not start work or normal activity again until at least a week after all the physical and mental symptoms of stress have gone.

2   When preparing to go back to work, go through your diary and cancel every engagement or meeting over the next six months that is not absolutely vital.

3   When you are able to start thinking clearly again,

consider what your priorities are and how you spend your time. List all your regular commitments, at home and work, and calculate the percentage of your time you give to each area of your life, such as:

- your important relationships

- caring for dependent relatives or friends

- your social life

- the clubs or societies you belong to

- the management of changes at home (e.g. moving house, building work, getting divorced, family weddings, bereavements)

- the activities of children or partners in which you are involved

Remember also to include:

- time for rest, exercise, relaxation and recreation

- time for work commitments

- unstructured time just for yourself

When you have worked out the percentage of time you normally give to each area, the figures may well be quite an eye-opener, showing quite clearly where the imbalance has crept in. Most people find work dominates the majority of their time and energy and causes the most stress. The other major cause is usually looking after other people's needs. But probably the main reason why most people get stressed is quite simply because they forget to put time aside for themselves. This leaves no time for rest, recuperation, reflection and creativity, or to process or 'digest' what is happening in life. Over time, failure to take time to be nourished and find meaning in life makes people very bored, unsatisfied, empty and depressed. To fill this sense of emptiness, people often use alcohol or drugs to make themselves feel better. Sometimes these difficult feelings cause people to give out even more to others, which drains them still further.

4. Re-organize your priorities, allocating the correct proportion of time to the key areas in your life.

The underlying essence of this process is to become clear again about your core values. The other vital element is to simplify life radically so that you bring real energy to the areas that matter to you. But the foundation stone to all of this is proper time for yourself, and this should appear at the top of your new list. Ideally, time for yourself should include totally unstructured time, as well as time to relax, meditate, exercise, and seek help from support groups, counsellors or complementary therapists. It should also include at least one creative activity. This may mean reviving an interest in art, music, literature, theatre or dance, for example. Creating unstructured time means leaving space for yourself each week just to potter, rest, reflect or read. If you live with others you must guard this space fiercely and get the people in your life to respect your special time alone. This may even encourage them to do the same.

Making time for yourself is a particularly helpful message and example to give children. Many adults programme their children for stress in later life. They organize their children's lives without leaving any space or 'down time' when they can be alone in their inner world. It then becomes increasingly hard for them to be on their own, which in turn is why so many adults find it difficult to be on their own and to develop a sustaining inner life. It is therefore important to start right from the beginning with children, allowing them space and time when they can literally unfold in their own creative, inner-directed way.

You will probably need to let go of as much as 50 per cent of all your other activities and projects. This may sound drastic, but half of the extra time you create by doing this will be for yourself, with the rest for doing properly the things you are committed to, without rush or struggle. It will also leave room for the inevitable growth of your activities. You may eventually have to do another major pruning exercise.

At work, reducing your goals by 50 per cent will take a great deal of clarity, courage and discipline. But taking the stress off yourself in this way will allow you in the end to achieve far better results on the projects you are working on. If this is simply impossible in your job, it may well be time for a change or to seriously challenge your managers about your job description. Usually, however, we are the ones who make our jobs impossible, by either being too ambitious or unrealistic, or by being incapable of saying no.

To combat severe stress you may need to challenge your belief that 'more is better'. Many of us think we will be considered virtuous or more lovable if we are high achieving. But the tendency to take on more and more can also be seen as a form of greed. It may look virtuous or altruistic but often it is driven, just like overeating, by an underlying hunger for more – in this case more power, money or recognition. These needs ultimately stem from an emotional or spiritual hunger that can be filled in far less destructive ways if emotional and spiritual needs are properly met. When addressing these underlying needs most people need counselling help.

If you are suffering from stress which is not so extreme, it is still important to get your own stress-reduction programme going. This should involve a mixture of relaxation and self-help techniques alongside your normal work. You can then slim down and re-prioritize your home, work and social activities in the same way as described above, making sure that there is plenty of time for you.

Sleep, rest and relaxation

To become really healthy and avoid cancer, addressing the need for proper sleep, rest and relaxation is vital. Sometimes, I like to think of life as being a bit like an infinity sign, imagining that we move outwards on one loop of the sign into activity, arousal and achievement, then flow back again in an equal and opposite loop into rest, relaxation, letting go and regeneration.

Sleep and rest

Indian Ayurvedic physicians believe that every day the body goes through a series of four-hourly cycles, starting at 2, 6 and 10 a.m. and 2, 6 and 10 p.m. At the end of the evening cycle, at 10 p.m., we naturally feel quite sleepy and ready to rest. However, if we resist this urge and stay up, we go into a new, more fiery type of energy cycle which will often keep us up late into the night. If we then need to get up early to work or look after children, we are literally 'burning the candle at both ends' and failing to get the restorative rest and sleep we need.

Many people do feel naturally sleepy around 9.30 to 10 p.m. and could easily go to bed then, but they overcome these feelings in order to try to achieve more and reduce their anxiety. In the Ayurvedic system, the best time to get up is soon after 6 a.m., with the light. Try to get your life more in harmony with these natural cycles of the body. Try also to make the cut-off point for all work-related activity the moment you walk through the door at home after work. If this is not possible, then make an absolute deadline of about 8 p.m., after which all time is spent relaxing and nourishing yourself in creative ways.

Start going to bed or settling down around 10 p.m. – whether this is to read, meditate, reflect, write down your feelings in a journal, or make love. All these things will deepen your connection with yourself and your loved ones. Make sure this gentle time is absolutely sacrosanct in your home life. Achieving this balance will make your life instantly richer and far healthier. Your immune system and tissue functioning will recover and the risk of cancer will diminish greatly.

Relaxation

Relaxing is something most of us have either forgotten how to do or never knew how to do in the first place. We have become used to feelings of pressure, anxiety and insecurity and, as a result, many people are very tense. As a doctor, when I ask people if they are able to relax, they often say 'Yes, I can relax really easily. All I have to do is close my eyes and I'm asleep straightaway.' But they do not realize sleep is not the same as relaxation.

In fact, people who go to sleep tense or anxious, often wake up just as anxious. This is because the body continues to make the stress chemicals adrenaline, noradrenaline and cortisol through the night. Consequently, people who go to sleep anxious, often have very anxious dreams, which can leave them feeling ragged and exhausted the next day.

If sleep does come the instant you close your eyes, it can mean you are actually exhausted, often because of stress. If this all sounds horribly familiar, you need to get yourself properly relaxed, either by consulting a relaxation therapist, yoga teacher, masseur or healer or using a relaxation tape. This will allow you to experience what it feels like to be deeply relaxed, and will show you what to aim for when doing relaxation exercises on your own.

Relaxation removes the effects of stress and fear from the body. It also helps the mind to start to unwind. When you start to do a relaxation exercise – with a relaxation therapist or on your own – first make yourself really comfortable and ensure you are not going to be disturbed. This means loosening tight clothing, taking off shoes, spectacles or tight jewellery, and making sure you can get into a comfortable reclined position, preferably with your feet level with or slightly above the head.

To begin with, it is best not to do relaxation exercises on your bed because you will probably go straight to sleep. You may also find that as you begin to relax properly you will feel chilly. It is therefore worth covering yourself with a light rug to prevent yourself from getting cold. Try, if you can, to unplug the telephone. Put a 'Do Not Disturb' sign on your door, or ask others not to interrupt you for at least half an hour. The next step is to settle into your position – sitting on a chair or sofa or lying on the floor – allowing yourself to feel very heavy and as if you have completely let go. A good relaxation therapist, teacher or tape will then usually invite you to consciously 'unplug' yourself from all your normal activities so that you can switch off completely for the next fifteen or twenty minutes.

Then start the relaxation exercise with three deep sighs or out breaths. Start first by breathing in deeply, as if right from the soles of your feet, and then breathe out, making an audible sighing sound as you do so. This gives an instant message to the body to let go. Thereafter, focus your attention on breathing, allowing the breath to deepen and the whole breathing pattern to relax. Once you have 'arrived' in this safe, cocooned space, go through each area of the body, releasing tension as you do so. Most people start at the top of the head and work downwards. So begin with the scalp, literally allowing it to relax and let go. From here, go one by one to the forehead, eyes, cheeks, mouth, tongue, jaw and throat, letting go of any tension you encounter.

Some people prefer to tense each area of the body as they come to it, actively squeezing the muscles tightly and then letting go. They find this makes it easier to focus on each area of the body. With either technique, attention then goes to the neck, shoulders, arms and chest. In the chest area, pay particular attention to the rib cage, allowing it to let go so that breathing can become deeper. Also pay special attention to the abdomen, where an enormous amount of tension and anxiety can be held in the solar plexus and surrounding musculature. Then move to the hips, pelvis, thighs, knees, calves, ankles and feet.

Theoretically, by the time you get to the tips of your toes, the whole body should be completely soft and relaxed. But in practice, if you are just starting to learn this technique, often by the time you get to your toes, the head and shoulders have tensed up again. It may therefore be worth repeating this whole exercise two or three times while you are learning to make sure you have fully let go throughout the whole body.

If you have achieved deep relaxation, either your body will feel very heavy or you will hardly be able to feel it at all. Our sense of position comes from nerve endings in the joints and balance receptors in the middle ear. If there is no movement in the body at all, as in a deep state of relaxation, we may temporarily lose the ability to tell where our body is. In this state, breathing should be very slow and shallow and the heart rate will also slow down. In stark contrast, when someone is stressed and feeling agitated mentally, the heart rate is rapid, possibly with palpitations, muscles are tense and breathing is irregular. People may even hold their breath when they are very anxious.

Once you have experienced deep relaxation and learnt to achieve this state on your own, it is then possible to start relaxing for twenty minutes a day at home (or even during a break at work). As people get more experienced at relaxing, they can stay relaxed for much longer. Most of us put far too much energy and effort into everything we do, getting more and more tense as we go along. When you have mastered relaxation, check every hour or so to see how much you have tensed up again. If you catch yourself feeling tense, try to let go of the tension in your shoulders, jaw and stomach, and to return breathing to a normal, deep, slow rate. Over time, a relaxed state will become the norm and feeling tense will become odd. Try to teach yourself the 'magic of minimal effort'. This means putting only the minimum effort required into all you do! You will soon find that you are doing less but achieving more.

Achieving and maintaining high energy levels

The importance of maintaining high energy levels and vitality was explained earlier under The Energy Model of Health. Eating well, exercising, resting and relaxing will all raise energy levels. But if you think your energy levels have dropped below the critical 30 per cent line, it is time to let go and allow them to be lifted for you through either healing or the energy medicines – shiatsu, acupuncture and homeopathy.

Healing

If you have never tried spiritual healing or are very sceptical, I urge you to give it a chance and try it for yourself. You do not need to be religious or to have faith for spiritual healing to work.

During healing, the healer meditates and, by placing his or her hands close to your body, becomes an 'energy channel'. This means the healer becomes a conduit for energy from higher sources – either a divine power or the life force of nature. It is impossible to say scientifically how this happens, but it quite definitely does. The resulting feeling is extremely nourishing and uplifting. Once they have tried healing, even people who were initially very suspicious cannot deny that it is a very lovely experience, and testify that the effects can make a real difference.

The beauty of healing is that you do not have to think, talk or do any work at all. The only requirement is be receptive to the healing energy. This is a bit like lying back and enjoying the sun or soaking in a warm bath. What is hard for many people, though, is the very idea of letting go and receiving from others. Such an admission of our vulnerability is difficult for us. In fact, many people in a depleted energy state try even harder to keep everything together, rather than resting and regenerating. If your energy levels have become very low, healing may be necessary two or three times a week until they rise to the point where you can begin to help yourself with yoga, tai chi, meditation, relaxation and exercise.

The energy medicines – shiatsu, acupuncture and homeopathy

Shiatsu and acupuncture are the traditional medicines of Japan and China respectively. In both systems, energy state is diagnosed by reading energy pulses. In acupuncture, pulses are taken at the wrist, and in shiatsu are taken in the abdomen or *hara*. With this information, a rebalancing of the body's energy can be carried out. In acupuncture this is done with needles, and in shiatsu, it is done with pressure from the fingers, hands or even elbows at pressure points throughout the body.

In the East it is said that traditionally people paid their acupuncturists while they were well and stopped if they became sick. For centuries these systems of medicine have been used primarily for prevention rather than treatment. This is an extremely useful attitude and behaviour for us to adopt in the West. An acupuncturist or shiatsu practitioner will quickly tell you what the underlying state of your energy is. You may need several sessions to get into a good state of balance, and once this has been achieved you may need to go monthly or every six weeks in order to maintain a high energy state and help prevent cancer.

Homeopathy also raises and balances the vital force but it is done through remedies given in tablet form, which interact with our own energy to optimize our state of health and vitality.

Working with your energy

Long term, the way to achieve optimum health and high energy levels is to be aware of what you do with your energy – how you spend it and how you build it. Most people are like a seriously overdrawn bank balance – they spend energy recklessly without a thought as to how they will replenish it. In fact, a tendency to overspend money often goes hand in hand with a tendency to overexpend energy. Overspending, like overeating, can be a compensation for emptiness inside, caused by failing to nourish ourselves emotionally and spiritually. Others find themselves depleted in energy because they simply don't have adequate support to cope with their commitments to children, elderly relatives, work and home life.

Begin to look at where you are expending or even haemorrhaging vital energy. Many of us spend vast amounts of energy getting caught up in the affairs of others or battling our way through the shops when they are crowded. We try to sustain crazy social or work lives and remain involved in extremely draining relationships. On a more subtle level, we may be living or working in places that literally drain our energy. Some people and places are like energy 'black holes' – even a telephone call with someone like this can leave us severely depleted. Or, as mentioned earlier, we may lose energy simply by putting too much energy into everything we do.

Some people are more energy sensitive than others. They are so tuned in to the energy of other people that they lose track of how they feel themselves. These energy-sensitive people can become 'symptom carriers' for their family or close friends since they are often very empathic types. They tend to keep soaking up difficult unharmonious energies around them in an attempt to re-equilibrate and harmonize the atmosphere. These people become particularly compromised if they fail to make space for themselves. If this describes you, make extra sure you spend plenty of time on your own, and around healthy energy. Learn to recognize people, places and activities which build your energy levels. People often say their energy levels are raised dramatically by trips to the country, gardens, forests, beauty, music and meditation, or quite simply by spending time alone either being still or in creative activity.

Once you start to think about it, you will begin to recognize exactly what feeds and drains your energy levels. You may find you are actually being propped up by the energy of another, perhaps because you are failing to take responsibility for building your own energy levels. It is important to change this pattern and raise your energy levels in a healthier way.

Try to make yourself a list of the things that feed and drain your energy. You could even do yourself a balance sheet and compare the debit and credit elements of your energy account. If it is clear that you are pouring your precious energy into many non-productive areas, then gradually start to eliminate the draining activities and replace them with things that lift your energy. This will overlap with your efforts to reduce stress, because cutting down planned activity, whether it is social or work, will also have a big effect on energy levels. But something that drains your energy is different from stress because certain situations or people can take a lot of your energy without you necessarily giving them much time. If, as well as re-prioritizing your time, you also start to avoid draining phone calls, difficult people, unnecessary shopping trips and other neurotic, non-productive behaviour, replacing all this 'doing' with simply 'being', your energy levels will rise dramatically.

Care must be taken over the issue of energy and exercise. Sometimes, exercising hard when you have little energy can reduce energy levels further. However, exercising when your energy levels are beginning to rise will strengthen you and raise your energy. It is a question of being aware of the effect exercise is having on your energy levels. This is also relevant to what has been said about resting – once you are more aware of what is going on with your underlying energy, you will stop overriding the signals from your body that you are tired and instead listen to your body and rest appropriately.

As energy levels rise there is an enhanced sense of intuition and connection with life, more synchronicity, or meaningful coincidences and heightened telepathic ability. This means that as energy levels rise, so does our state of consciousness. Most important, though, people feel happier, more confident and in control, and more able to live meaningful, creative lives.

Cancer is much less likely to develop when the body is in a high-energy state. It has been shown that in those with higher energy, immune and enzyme activity increases at cell level. High energy literally wakes up the body's tissues and defence mechanisms. This makes cell nuclei far less likely to mutate, but if they do they are quickly picked up and eradicated from the body.

Being excited, enthusiastic and passionate about life has the most profound effect on energy and vitality. When we suddenly find love, become fully expressed in our work or open the door to our spirituality, energy levels can jump right off the graph.

Calming your mind with meditation

When Zoe Lindgren was diagnosed with cancer she was pregnant with her second child. Doctors advised her to terminate the pregnancy. But Zoe, who was thirty-one at the time, refused. Six months into the pregnancy, she had a lumpectomy to remove the cancerous growth, and after her daughter was born she underwent radiotherapy.

As soon as Zoe was diagnosed with cancer, she went to the Bristol Cancer Help Centre. Because she had cared for her mother with cancer, she was already aware of the Centre's work. The main change she made at this point was to become a vegetarian.

Two years later, in 1991, she was diagnosed with cancer again, but this time it was in her lungs and lymph system. Zoe was told that even with chemotherapy she had only a maximum of eighteen months to live. While undergoing chemotherapy she felt at her lowest ebb, and it became of paramount importance to her that she regain control of what was a very out of control situation. She was determined not to become a victim and wanted to make the experience as positive as she could. After four of six chemotherapy treatment sessions, she could take no more. She ended conventional medicine and turned instead to complementary therapies to help her confront her illness, mental state and lifestyle.

Zoe recognized immediately that the really big problem she had to tackle was her pressured lifestyle and the stress levels she engendered as a successful architect. She knew that if her body was to survive it was vital to calm her mind, so she embarked on a concentrated programme of mind–body techniques, favouring particularly meditation and visualization. To begin with, she found the new regime an uphill struggle. But with the guidance and support of the Bristol Cancer Help Centre, she was able to master these techniques. She also had acupuncture, homeopathy, healing and reflexology, and found emotional support for her husband, Andy, too. She learnt through counselling about being non-judgmental, how to look at the positive side of things, and about the harmful effects on the body of a negative self-image.

But the most important thing of all, she feels, was her decision to leave her pressured 'life in the fast lane' to go and live in a forest in Wales. Since making this move Zoe has become a completely different woman. The combination of her peaceful home, daily meditations and healthy diet has turned her into a radiant picture of health and she now positively emanates health, well-being and tranquillity.

Ten years later, at forty-three, Zoe is still cancer-free, and is now working part-time as a reflexologist. While she is sure the chemotherapy and tamoxifen she took in 1991 'doused the fire' of the disease, she has outlived her prognosis by years and has clearly achieved a most remarkable recovery. She has done everything in her power to prevent the disease recurring and has achieved an absolutely outstanding stabilization of her condition.

Zoe now has a much better quality of life than ever before and feels her greatest achievement has been the development of her inner strength and peace of mind. Her success is an enormous testimony to the power of the holistic approach to health and is a fitting reward for all the hard work she has put into her recovery process. Zoe's story clearly demonstrates the need, above all others, to reduce our stress levels and achieve inner peace if we want to get well and stay well.

The single most beneficial thing you can do to revolutionize your health is to start meditating. This will make every other aspect of your life easier. As you become calmer with a clearer state of mind, your energy levels will quickly rise. Resistance and inertia will melt away and it will become easier to put all other aspects of life on a healthier footing. Neuroses will lose their grip and you will once again able to see the wood for the trees.

It is important to say here that learning to meditate does not involve becoming part of a sect or taking up a religion. You can meditate in a religious context, within Buddhism, say, but it is equally possible to meditate without any religion or belief system at all.

Meditation is a process of calming the mind, so that people can experience pure consciousness and the connection between their consciousness and all that is around them. Most people go through life without ever experiencing this clear state of mind. Instead, they are totally preoccupied with what goes on in their minds and their sense of separation from everything and everybody else. Most of us believe we are our thoughts, feelings, sensations and emotions, but actually these things are the contents of our consciousness rather than our consciousness itself.

When we learn how to still our minds and get untangled from the contents of consciousness, we will discover that the natural underlying state of our consciousness is one of bliss. This is why all the religious texts of the world say that the kingdom of heaven is within. As soon as this still and open state of mind is discovered, people quickly realize it feels better than much of the external stimulation they seek. As a result, their continual quest for external satisfaction diminishes and their inner state becomes greatly enriched. Although people will still need to fulfil their potential in life, this is likely to happen in a far more gentle, wholesome and satisfying manner.

Psychologically, the great benefit of meditation is that emotions begin to settle and people become more sensitive to their own inner voice or wisdom. This wise part of ourselves will often know exactly what we need or don't need in any given situation. As people base their lives more and more on the wisdom of this inner-knowing or higher self, a lot of problems or neurotic behaviour will simply dissolve away.

Physiologically what is happening is that the chaotic beta waves associated with intense mental activity and stress are replaced with gentler alpha waves. At deeper levels of mediation these can be replaced by very slow delta or even theta waves. When this happens, the neuro-peptide cocktail in the body is changed entirely and tissues and cells begin to function optimally.

All meditators report a wonderfully enhanced sense of living in harmony with nature, and feel supported by life rather than constantly struggling against it. Their sense of separation and isolation is diminished, eventually replaced with a wonderful sense of connection to life and a feeling of being part of the whole. However, many people are addicted to their chaos and 'emotional drama' and will resist attempts to quieten down emotionally. But once the addiction to pain and emotional drama is replaced with real joy, a much deeper and more satisfying sense of emotional fulfilment and pleasure can be attained.

In relation to cancer, meditation alone has been shown to heal the disease. This is demonstrated by the work in Australia of Ainsley Mearess, who took people with cancer into prolonged states of meditation. In many cases the deep calming and reactivation of the immune system led to quite extraordinary remission and healing – powerful proof of the connection between mind and body. There are some who say the cellular chaos of cancer is a reflection of our mental and emotional chaos. And it may be that until we sort out our collective fear and dishar-mony, we will never be able to eradicate cancer. I am sure there is a great deal of truth in this, because of the

profound effects of our state of mind on tissue functioning. That is why I believe meditation holds the most
potential for turning around our susceptibility to cancer.

Learning meditation

There are many ways to learn meditation. The practice
always involves focusing attention on a single thing until
the mind becomes so still that it transcends even that
focus. This can be a sound – or mantra as it is called in
yogic practice – repeated in your head. It can be a visual
object or picture such as a mandala – an image which
draws your focus to its centre. Or you can keep your attention fixed on the flow of your breathing. Other forms of
meditation involve focusing on loving feelings in your
heart and on generating feelings of love for yourself and
the rest of humanity and the world. Some traditions focus
on the sensation of the skin. This technique is often used
in Vipassana meditation.

The best-known school of meditation, using a mantra
technique, is Transcendental Meditation (TM), and this
is a highly effective way of learning the skill (see
Appendix 1). Focusing on the breath is often associated
with yogic and Buddhist practices, and teachers can be
found through the British Wheel of Yoga and Friends of
the Western Buddhist Order as well as other schools of
meditation (see Appendix 1).

For most Westerners, learning to meditate is difficult
because we have such busy minds and have never learnt
how to still them. In order to master the technique, the
essence therefore has to be adequate tuition and regular
practice. Joining a regular meditation class or group is

highly recommended until you are able to meditate for at least twenty minutes a day at home by yourself. Initially, meditating in a group will make the whole thing far easier, for the stillness and peace generated by the group will be catching. Whatever else you do as a result of reading this book, I urge you most strongly to develop a meditation practice. This will undoubtedly unlock your ability to make the right steps towards health, well-being and fulfilment in all areas of your life.

CHAPTER 5:
WORKING WITH THE
MIND–BODY–SPIRIT
CONNECTION

The most profound difference you can make to your health is to attend to the underlying state of your spirit. You can do this directly with meditation but you can also do it by unburdening your spirit and moving towards a lifestyle which expresses and nourishes you. This will enable you to become truly well, from the inside out. When you are at peace with yourself, living authentically, fully engaged with life in a meaningful and exciting way, the reverberations of this extremely wholesome feeling will affect the way every tissue and cell of your body functions, and you will become healthy and alive.

Here are two really good examples of the changes in health which can occur when people start to live in ways that are true to themselves. The first concerns a patient of the brilliant dermatologist Dr Ann McGuire, who became renowned for her unique approach to skin problems, working with the mind–body connection. The basic premise of her work is that 'the skin is the mirror of the psyche'. One day, at the end of a long hard clinic, a man came in who had had severe psoriasis for many years. He had come expecting an in-depth exploration of the emotional side of his skin problem. But instead he found an irritable, tired Ann who had simply run out of steam.

When he asked the doctor what was wrong with him, she replied: 'It's quite simple – you are in the wrong place, at the wrong time, doing the wrong thing with your life.' With this she closed his file and told him she could give him no more time. Later on, she felt absolutely dreadful about having treated this poor man so dismissively, and was quite worried about the repercussions she might have to face. So when she saw his name on her clinic list a few months later, she was sure he was going to be extremely angry with her. But this couldn't have been further from the truth! He bounded into the room and practically kissed her. She quickly realized that his psoriasis had gone altogether. She asked him what on earth had happened and he said:

> Well, of course, you were completely right – I was in the wrong place, at the wrong time, doing the wrong thing with my life. For twenty years, I had been farming and slaughtering animals for meat. Running the abattoir had actually been distressing me deeply. Over the years I became more and more revolted by the whole process, but was unable to face getting rid of it and starting again in a new direction. When you said that, the whole thing came into focus for me and that same afternoon I put my

business on the market. It sold within a month and I am now in the process of turning my land over to crop farming. The minute I made the decision, it was as if a huge weight had been lifted off my shoulders. The relief was immense, and almost immediately the psoriasis started to shift. Now, for the first time in years, my skin is clear!

So from having started the consultation a very worried woman, Ann ended up celebrating with this man the powerful shift he had made in his life and health.

The second illustration comes from the area of cancer medicine, and is a good example of the work of Dr Lawrence LeShan, one of the founders of the holistic health and mind–body medicine movement. Larry worked with cancer patients for many years, trying to help them get their lives back on track in order to help heal their disease. In this case it was a friend called Peter, who was very ill with a serious pancreatic tumour. He had been told he had just weeks to live. Peter was in hospital when Larry saw him, jaundiced and plugged into a drip, looking pretty ghastly and extremely depressed.

Larry started off down his normal track, asking Peter what it was in life that really excited and motivated him. Knowing Larry well, Peter replied: 'For goodness sake, Larry, can't you see, I'm dying! This is no time to talk about what turns me on!' But Larry gently persisted, and after an hour or so ascertained that Peter's true passion was sculpture. However, the profession he had ended up following all his life, due to parental pressure, was architecture.

He had been a good and successful architect, but had

never felt truly excited by his work. Larry asked him where, in an ideal world, he would have liked to do his sculpture. Peter said, 'Florence, of course!' Mischievously, taking a gamble, Larry said to him, 'If I turned up here with a ticket to Florence and an opportunity to do some sculpture there, would you take it?' Peter sat bolt upright and said, 'Of course I would! What have I got to lose? I'm just sitting here waiting to die.' This was all the encouragement Larry needed. He went off and arranged, with Peter's family, to get a ticket, and he found a sculpting course which was starting shortly in Florence.

Within a week Peter suddenly found himself in Florence, where he set up a small studio. He was weak but his excitement and sense of anticipation were immense. He not only started and completed the six-month sculpting course, but also fell in love while he was in Florence. He went on to have an absolutely enchanting two years there, exploring his new relationship, his life passion of sculpting and the wonderful museums and buildings of the city. At the end of this two years, he was called back to America on family business. Within three months of leaving Italy, his cancer returned with a vengeance. He died peacefully at home, three weeks later.

Peter died a very happy, grateful and satisfied man. He had allowed his spirit to fly free for two glorious years and, as tough as it was to let go into death after having known such sweetness, he had been able to let go gracefully in the knowledge that, even if only for two years, he had been fully alive.

In the first of these cases, it was the release from terrible inner conflict that allowed the physical healing to occur. In the second, it was only when Peter became fully authentic and truly expressed that his immune system kicked in again and stabilized the tumour. These cases illustrate just how profound is the connection between our mind, body and spirit, and how crucial it is to attend to how happy and fulfilled we are if we really want to be well and prevent cancer.

ATTENDING TO THE STATE OF YOUR SPIRIT

Attending to your spirit has three main phases. The first is the *unburdening* phase. You need to unburden yourself of:

- emotions you have been carrying long term.

- disabling attitudes or limiting beliefs you have picked up earlier in life.

- roles you play or personas you project which do not represent who you really are.

- dominating presences or forces in your life.

The second phase involves *discovering who you really are*. This whole process could be described as 'becoming true to yourself'. It entails:

- eliciting your core values in life (particularly what it is that gives your life purpose or meaning).

- finding ways to express yourself in the world (with

respect to your job, the environment in which you live, the relationships you choose, your sexuality and so on, as well as the more obvious outlets you may have for your creative and physical energies).

In essence, this is all about you – the unique being that you are – being enabled and empowered to reach your full potential. It has absolutely nothing to do with competitiveness, though; it is about allowing yourself to flourish and grow and to express your true nature, irrespective of anyone else.

The third area is *attending to your spiritual nourishment*. This may be through:

- beauty, art or fine music

- religion

- meditation

- spiritual retreats

- developing your personal spirituality

- dedicated service to others

- sharing the spontaneous fun and creativity of children

- creative activity

- giving and receiving love

But being able to do any of this is based first and foremost on being prepared to develop a healthy relationship with yourself.

DEVELOPING A HEALTHY RELATIONSHIP WITH YOURSELF

If you are already able to look after yourself well, the advice given here does not apply to you. However, this is a rarity! Sadly, most of us are pretty hopeless at looking after ourselves properly. We are usually at the bottom of the list of people and things we look after. As I said before, we usually take far better care of our cars and homes than ourselves – being careful to get cars serviced regularly and houses redecorated. Perhaps, if people were forced to have yearly MOTs, they would not neglect themselves so badly.

By answering the following questions, you will get a basic idea of what your relationship with yourself is like.

- Do you eat properly?

- Do you get enough sleep?

- Do you exercise regularly?

- Do you walk away from abusive relationships?

- Do you look after your appearance?

- Do you stay out of debt?

- Do you refrain from abusing or harming yourself physically and mentally?

- Do you believe you are valuable?

- Do you believe you deserve attention, love, money and nice possessions?

- Do you believe you are lovable?
- Are you able to spend time alone?
- Do you give yourself time for rest and recuperation?

  And, most importantly of all:

- Do you love, or even like yourself?

If most of the answers to these questions are yes, your relationship with yourself is in pretty good shape. But if there are a lot of no answers, then your relationship with yourself could probably do with a great deal of improvement. People who do not have a good relationship with themselves and do not value themselves properly have low self-esteem. In this situation, people are unlikely to put in place, let alone maintain, activities which allow them to fulfil themselves, and it will be difficult to implement any of the advice in this book. So the first step in your resurrection and cancer-prevention programme is to set about changing your relationship with yourself.

The relationship we have with ourselves is usually based on the relationship we had with our parents, or significant adults, in childhood. If we have been loved, cherished, nurtured and encouraged, we will probably be good at doing this for ourselves. If, on the other hand, we have been neglected, criticized, abandoned, abused and shown very little encouragement or affection, this is likely to be the way we will treat ourselves too. But it is possible to change the relationship with yourself and begin treating yourself properly. More often than not, though, it takes the experience of a new kind of nurturing relationship with another to reset the template. This is where counselling, psychotherapy, healing and the complementary therapies that employ touch can be extremely helpful.

All these emotional and physical therapies are based on treating the client with what is known as 'unconditional positive regard'. This means the relationship is based on non-judgmental, loving kindness and care and concern for the client. All holistic therapies have at their root the aim of enabling you to develop this sort of relationship with yourself so that when the period of therapy is over you can take up this nurturing process for yourself. Once this caring relationship has been modelled for you, you will be able, bit by bit, to take over and start giving yourself what it is you really need.

If you feel your self-esteem is very low, you should probably go for counselling or psychotherapy. It is terribly important to have an introductory meeting to make sure the therapist is suitable for you, rather than the other way round. If this experience is to build your self-esteem and confidence, you must feel entirely comfortable with this person and feel he or she has genuine warmth towards you. Have no hesitation whatsoever in meeting two or three therapists before you make your choice.

If you think you can build a new relationship with yourself without this kind of help, the golden rules are:

1 Learn to put yourself at the top of the list of people to look after. If you look after yourself properly, you will be in better shape to care for others and will be giving them a terrific model to follow and apply in

their own lives. You will also have a much healthier relationship with your partner. When you are able to care for yourself properly, you will be far less needy and therefore far less likely to stay with unsuitable partners, because you will not be so dependent on the 'crumbs from their table'.

2   Get to know yourself and your needs well. Get used to tuning in to how you feel, and react appropriately. This means listening to your body's needs, for food, sleep, sex, and exercise; to your emotional needs, for comfort, warmth and support, and to the needs of your soul or spirit for peace, space or adventure.

3   Learn to express your feelings and ask clearly for what you need (without getting upset if the answer is no!). If this is very hard for you, take a course in assertiveness to learn how to communicate your needs without fear, and to accept a 'no' without taking it as a rejection.

4   Work through the questions at the beginning of this section, making sure you are looking after yourself properly in all of these ways.

The above advice is mainly for people who are very 'other centred' and may have a negative self-image and poor self-esteem. But sometimes the reverse is the problem. If you have become rather self-centred, you need to move in the other direction and learn to think and care more about the needs of others, as well as your own. Generally speaking, though, it is better to err on the side of being self-centred, because people are far more likely to take good care of themselves if they have a high opinion of themselves.

Having a good relationship with yourself can be described as being your own 'good parent'. You cease to be at the mercy of your needy, greedy, demanding, anarchic inner child and are instead able to give yourself what will sustain, nourish and develop you long term. This means acquiring a more mature sense of what you really need, rather than always going for 'instant gratification' or what feels good at the time. This is not to diminish the value of spontaneity or giving yourself treats, but it is important to know the difference between treats which will genuinely nurture you and those which will give you a boost now but cost you later.

In the transpersonal model of psychology, these different aspects of ourselves are seen as sub-personalities, whose needs have to be negotiated. As you become increasingly self-aware, many sub-personalities may emerge that you can work with, recognize and cater for.

Changing your relationship with yourself does not happen overnight. But, as with everything else, having the intention to learn how to be gentler, more loving, more permissive and more responsible towards yourself, is a strong starting point. See if you can make this commitment to yourself now, before you go on to read how to make practical steps to improve the state of your spirit. Once again, it may be a good idea to make notes of the areas in which you wish to make changes in your life.

UNBURDENING THE SPIRIT

Letting go of emotions

The holistic concept that 'what the mind represses, the body expresses' has already been mentioned. Many people, however, are simply too scared to express their feelings, but these feelings have to go somewhere. A feeling produces chemical neuropeptides in the brain and body, and as feelings are expressed, these neuropeptides are discharged or metabolized, and equilibrium is restored. (Neuropeptides released in tears of rage, by the way, are completely different to those found in tears of grief or heartbreak.) But should these chemicals not be released, they become stuck in the body, causing physiological change. Dr Candace Pert, who helped to discover these chemicals, called them 'molecules of emotion' (see Books in Appendix 1).

It is useful to define our 'feelings' as what we feel when something happens. When feelings are not expressed and turn into memories in the mind and body, they become emotions which can be retained long term. Sometimes, people are quite comfortable expressing one kind of feeling, but not another. For example, some of us find it easy to cry, but are never able to get angry. In others, it is the reverse – they will erupt like a volcano but would rather kill themselves than cry in public!

The most common feelings people hang on to are grief, disappointment, bitterness, guilt and anger. When these become lodged as emotions in the body, they can have particular effects on different organs. For example, grief often tends to affect the lungs and throat; anger effects the liver and gut; bitterness the pancreas; disappointment the kidneys, and guilt the nervous system. These are very broad generalizations, often observed through Oriental energy medicines, but in practice it is surprising how often these general rules are true. All of these effects occur through PNI or mind–body mechanisms.

The other major effect of these emotions is on the blood and immune systems. It has already been mentioned that stress and upset reduce the number of circulating immune cells and also make them less active, as well as decreasing the amount of oxygen carried in the haemoglobin of red blood cells. If you are burdened with a lot of old emotion from upsets, losses or frustration in the past, then it is an extremely good idea, both for the health of your immune system and for your ultimate protection against cancer, to offload it. This can be done in many ways. The most common way is through counselling or psychotherapy, when a person is taken right into a particular emotional memory and allowed, in a variety of ways, to discharge the energy or emotion felt at the time, and to which they are still holding on or embodying. Another route can be through the body. Good-quality massage or shiatsu, and powerful sex will often touch into old emotion, which can then be expressed if support is there. Spiritual healing can also unlock these doors and allow emotion to flow.

Another way involves being helped to actively forgive and let go of old hurts or wounds. People often hang on to or even nurse old grievances, even bearing grudges and resentments against people who have died. This is clearly not a good way to be. Not only do we become silted up with these harmful emotions, but part of our vital energy is trapped and inaccessible to us for living. Some therapists or group workers will concentrate on this forgiveness route. There are many groups, classes and opportunities for self-development work which focus on this area of healing the past (see Appendix 1).

Changing difficult attitudes and limiting beliefs

As well as forming the basis of the relationship with ourselves, early life is also the source of many underlying attitudes and beliefs about life and our abilities. When we are children we are very trusting and tend to believe what adults tell us. We are also equally affected by what they fail to tell us. If we get the message that we are not good enough, this will become our belief and, as adults, we will tend to give up even trying to get the things we want. If we do not get the attention and encouragement we need, we will believe we are unlovable and constantly strive for approval and attention.

If our environment as a child has been hostile and abusive, we tend to believe the world is a very dangerous place and are driven constantly by a sense of fear and insecurity (even if, to others, our situation seems quite secure). If we have had a harsh, critical, judgmental parent figure, we are often very harsh and judging of ourselves. If we have been told that children should be seen and not heard, it becomes difficult for us to be spontaneous or exuberant. If we have been told off every time we got angry or cried, then it will be extremely difficult to express emotion. If we have discovered that the way to get attention is by being sexually provocative, we may be sexually manipulative as adults.

Whilst these survival codes may have worked in childhood, they may when we are adults severely limit our pleasure, fulfilment and ability to reach our potential. Worse still people can pick up the message that they do not really deserve good things to happen to them and so would rather push good things away than endure the discomfort of receiving. Often people who overgive have this underlying belief. Although they are very generous themselves, if you try to give them anything they find it almost impossible to accept. Most of us are stuffed full of limiting beliefs – that we cannot have the love, money, power or enjoyment that we really want and need – and as a result live in a semi-depressed state all of our lives.

To turn this situation around, start to identify what underlying attitudes are affecting your behaviour or curbing your expectations, and replace them with much healthier ones. This kind of work can be done with a transpersonal counsellor (see Appendix 1). Once you start looking, it is quite easy to unearth these beliefs. The way to replace them is, first and foremost, to challenge yourself every time you find these attitudes coming into play. The other way is to make a list of your attitudes and limiting beliefs, and then make a separate set of statements which reverse them. For example, if you believe 'I am unlovable', write on a clean piece of paper 'I am lovable'. If you believe 'I do not deserve to be wealthy', write on the new list, 'I deserve wealth and abundance in my life'. Once you have made a list of reverse statements, you can use them as affirmations and repeat them to yourself on a regular basis. You can also repeat and affirm the healthy belief to yourself whenever you find an old, limiting belief is 'running you' in a given situation.

By doing this you will replace, over time, the negative messages of your upbringing with positive messages and beliefs. Eventually, you will be able to behave according to this new code and not the old one. It is much easier to do this work with a therapist than on your own. But it is certainly not impossible to do it yourself, especially if you keep a journal and add to the list when you discover new ways in which you are limiting or compromising yourself.

Shedding unhelpful roles and personas

Our roles or personas in adult life are also an extension of the attitudes and beliefs we have adopted from childhood. For example, if the desire to win approval has extended into your professional life, you may have chosen a well-respected role such as that of doctor, nurse, vet or vicar. If you have grown up believing the world is a very frightening place, you may have built your life around trying to take control of others by becoming a politician, teacher, policeman or member of the armed forces. This is not to say being a carer, politician or policeman is not the perfect role in life for some people. But it will largely depend on whether you are doing this

job from your strength or weakness, from your whole-
ness or your wound (or 'shadow', as it is known in
Jungian psychology).

The simple questions to ask yourself here are:

- Does my role genuinely reflect who I am, giving me
  excitement, life and energy?

- Is my role driven by my underlying fear or the secondary gains the role brings with it?

An example of a role or persona which is 'shadow' driven
would be the seemingly generous person who is actually
giving out a great deal because of his own immense emptiness and need. By behaving in this way, he is really trying
to show other people how he would like to be treated
himself but is too scared to ask. By overgiving he will
become even more depleted and is likely, ultimately, to
go into some form of burn-out or depression. This has its
foundations in the anger he feels inside at not being
treated properly.

Again, it is easier to examine these things with a therapist rather than on your own. A very useful way of
looking at your roles, personas or sub-personalities is to
attend the six introductory workshops run by the Centre
for Transpersonal Psychology (see Appendix 1). In doing
this you will get a good 'map' of your psyche and the
characters which inhabit it. You can learn which are your
dominant sub-personalities and which hardly ever see the
light of day. Sometimes, one of the sub-personalities
which has been submerged by the others can feel much
closer to the real you. Your true happiness may depend

upon allowing this aspect of yourself to develop and come forwards.

A good example of this comes from a colleague of mine who had breast cancer. At the time she was a school-teacher and 'executive wife', producing endless immaculate dinner parties for her husband's high-powered business associates. In a period of soul-searching after being diagnosed, she realized that none of this was really her and that, at heart, she was really a 'creative' who adored nature and natural medicine. Over time, she gradually withdrew from her former roles and allowed the gentler aspect of her personality to emerge. She now lives as a potter, organic gardener and spiritual healer, and is radiantly well twenty years after her initial diagnosis with breast cancer!

If you try to identify your sub-personalities yourself, 'go inside' and conjure up in your mind's eye all the different aspects of yourself. Some will be obvious, others may be fainter but nonetheless very important. Maybe you are a combination of a bossy headmistress or headmaster, slave driver, old gardener, opera singer, striptease artist and Mother Teresa! Try to get a sense of which of your sub-personalities really serve and express you well, and which give you the greatest energy. Compare this with the ones which compromise and drain you. If you are not satisfied with the ways things are, ask yourself whether it might not be time to start moving towards expressing one of your less dominant aspects which would serve you better and make your life a happier place.

Getting free of dominant presences or forces

Another reason why people fail to express themselves properly is that somebody or something is dominating them to such an extent they don't know how they feel or what they want. We talk about being 'possessed' by the dead, but it is also possible to be 'possessed' or dominated by the living! People who were completely dominated as children by the emotional needs of their parents or siblings are often, as a result, permanently in reaction to the state or needs of other family members. This can also happen in school or at work, when a dominant character constantly organizes all the attention around him- or herself, manipulating you in the process.

This often happens in partnerships too, where one person's needs are always dominant over the other's. Of course, powerful, needy parents can continue to dominate the lives of their offspring until a ripe old age if this pattern is not challenged and broken early on. When such a pattern is set early, it is quite hard to break. Should you be in this position, your later relationships may well be chosen on the basis of finding someone else to take on this dominating role in your life, since this way of being has become your 'comfort zone' – albeit an undermining situation for you. The problem is, when you are being dominated in this way, it is very hard to know yourself well and what your needs really are.

Extensions of this phenomenon can be found at many different levels. For example, we are all dominated by the high-tech, marketing-led world in which we live, which

itself is dominated by materialistic values. We are dominated by left-brain, achievement-orientated education
systems. We are dominated by reductionistic medicine!
Those of a gentler, more spiritual nature, often find themselves 'on the back foot', somewhat overwhelmed by these
types of societal pressure. It is difficult for them to assert
their own values and lifestyle, and this may lead to chronic
compromise at many levels of life.

If people are very sensitive, the atmosphere or energy
of a building or the area in which they live may dominate them too. There can also be problems if people are
forced to live in a country with a culture which is very
different to their own, where the dominant values all
around them are in conflict with their own underlying
values or nature.

Without realizing it, we may be using a lot of energy
to resist the dominant forces around us. The key here is
to recognize the phenomenon in the first place. The
minute you become aware that you are 'in the power' of
another person, value system, situation or place, you can
begin to do something about it.

The other aspect of this dynamic is that very often
those who allow themselves to be dominated can in other
circumstances be very dominant. In the extreme, this can
mean that people who have been abused can become
abusers themselves. To make this realization can be shat-
tering, and it often requires a therapist's help to get out
of this cycle. If you have been abused long term it
may take a while to rebuild your sense of yourself
once you are no longer being dominated. However, once
embarked upon, this process of 'reclaiming your power'

will enrich and strengthen you and eventually give you an enormous sense of relief. This in turn will mean your energy and will are no longer sapped and you will have much stronger resources for your own healing and self-defence.

RE-ORIENTATION TO YOUR TRUE SELF

Almost inevitably, as you stop being the way other people want you to be, the question arises, 'Who is the real me?' You may never have had a chance in your whole life to think about this question. People are constantly on the receiving end of pressure from parents, teachers and society to live up to their expectations, to be the way they want them to be, to take 'good' advice or simply to 'play the game'.

Discovering your core values

To find out what for you would be a fully authentic life, it is a good idea to take some quiet reflective time in a loving, supportive environment. This could be in retreat, in a therapeutic group, or with good friends who are aware you need time and space to re-orientate yourself. Start by doing a relaxation exercise and then focus your attention on your heart area. Concentrate on generating loving feelings in the heart, towards someone close to you or to yourself, or a more generalized sense of compassion towards others. When you are in this loving 'heart space' ask yourself:

- What is most important to me in life?
- What really matters to me?

  and then note down your responses.

Repeating this exercise several times on different days is a good idea. You will probably find that as the days pass you make an archaeological journey through deeper and deeper levels of yourself, until eventually you discover your innermost values. If this does not come easily to you, you could try imagining you have been diagnosed with a threatening illness and have been told you have only a year to live. Then ask yourself what would be really important to you, and what you would want to do with your time and energy in this remaining year. Imagining this has a tendency to sharpen the focus of the mind greatly!

Checking your will to live

After looking more deeply within yourself, you may find that you are not really that keen to go on living at all. A big part of you may even be longing for death. Don't be afraid if you discover this. Freud asserted that all of us have equal and opposite urges – Thanetos, the urge towards death, and Eros, the urge towards life. Normally, people move backwards and forwards between these poles, but some of us have a much stronger longing for death than others. Other people are so frightened of dying that an enormous amount of their energy is taken up trying to avoid even thinking about death, even if, underneath, they have lost their will to live.

Therefore, as a way of developing a far deeper relationship with yourself, it can be very helpful to examine your feelings about death and dying to discover where your true motivation lies. It is said people can only truly embrace life and live it to the full when they can also embrace the reality of death, and when the desire for death has been worked through to a point where they can genuinely make a choice for life.

Most people working in the holistic field view death not as 'failure' or even necessarily the end, but more as a transition. When you are working in this profound territory, it is good to ask yourself if you really do have the will to live or whether it has been beaten or squashed out of you by life's difficulties. If you are ambivalent about life, are deeply soul weary or just plain lost, it may well be time to seek a combination of spiritual healing and transpersonal psychotherapy to help you rekindle your commitment to life and find joy in living.

If you find out that your main purpose for living is your children or partner, then it may be worth exploring further to see whether there are unexpressed areas of yourself which need to emerge. These areas may have been abandoned as your life has become focused on other things. Whilst dedication to our nearest and dearest is absolutely right and wonderful, living out your life through others is not a good way to be. It can make you very dependent on them and them on you, and make it harder for them to have their own lives.

Living life with purpose and meaning

Once you have a clear sense of what really matters and excites you in life, the task then is to make sure this is reflected in the way you spend your time. If the very best bit of your life is squashed into a tiny fraction of your time, the soul or spirit will inevitably suffer. Once you know where your priorities lie, try step by step to change the balance in your life and watch your health and happiness blossom as you become more and more alive.

Jung, one of the most significant psychologists of recent times, said there is one state above all others which will surely kill a man – living life without meaning. For some, this sense of meaning will come through their inner life, their creativity or their relationship to the Divine. For others, it will be from a concrete focus such as helping to rehouse the homeless or feed the starving.

Increasingly, people are finding meaning in their lives through trying to understand and become conscious of the journey through life of their soul or spirit. People with a spiritual orientation often see themselves as 'spiritual beings in physical bodies'. Whilst anticipating their ultimate release back into the spiritual dimension at the time of death, they seek to understand the purpose of their incarnation and try to heed the lessons they are taught as they progress along life's path. This is consistent with the Eastern view of continuous reincarnation into different lifetimes until we have learnt enough not to need to come back any more.

Whatever your belief, the important thing for the immune system is to be as happy, excited and committed as possible in life. Lawrence LeShan described this as 'singing your own song' – feeling full of excitement when you wake each day and full of gratitude as you go to sleep. For many people this is a very long way from how they currently are. Our goal must be to seek this kind of happiness – breaking where necessary the addiction we have to our suffering and the comfort of staying stuck in our safe but unsatisfying rut.

Self-expression

One of the great 'soul' needs is for self-expression and for recognition of who we are. We are all unique and different, and encouraging our own personal forms of expression is fundamental for both individual health and the health of society. Unfortunately, the Victorian ethos and schooling most of us received tends to encourage the reverse, squashing individuality and encouraging uniformity. Educational processes by and large tend to push children and students through the same courses, so that they achieve the same standards in the same subjects at the same age. At the age of fifteen we are allowed to make some choices as we lean towards different career paths, but it is estimated that by this point the school system has lost the interest of about six out of seven children. This is because the way we are taught at school is only one of seven key learning styles. The vast majority of children going through the school system will never come anywhere near reaching their potential or being able to express themselves well in life.

It is very important for health to redress the inhibiting influences of our schooling, and to make strenuous efforts in all other areas of society to reverse this trend too. It is important at school, at home, at work and in the community to enjoy the differences in people and the unique skills they bring to situations. Most particularly, we must learn not to be prejudiced and discriminating towards people who do not take the conventional path. For yourself, check you are expressing your true self in the job you choose, the place in which you live, the people with whom you maintain relationships, and in your sexuality, creativity, physicality and appearance.

If you dress to please others, stop immediately and start dressing in a way that you like. If you make love in a way you think is expected of you or that your partner likes, think again and start finding how you would like to express yourself sexually. If you live in a house which is full of your parents' old furniture, in an area you don't like, think again about where and how you would like to live. If you have inherited a lot of your parents' things, you might find it amazingly refreshing to get rid of the history you are dragging around with you.

Start defining your own taste, hanging on to only one or two key things for historic and sentimental value. If you are a very physical person who loves to dance, run or climb mountains, but have forgone these pursuits as you got older, get going again and get your body moving.

If you feel limited or inhibited in your relationships, make a stand to change the relationship pattern so you can be exactly the way you are. If not, the other person will usually be aware you are not being yourself and will lose respect for you. There is nothing more off-putting than somebody who is inauthentic in this way. If someone doesn't like or want to be with the real you, then it is definitely time to leave the relationship anyway.

If you feel too vulnerable to let go of a 'false' relationship, seek the support of a counsellor to help you through the transition period. On the other hand, if it is a long-term committed relationship you are in, then seeking counselling yourself or jointly with your partner through the relationship counselling charity Relate (see Appendix 1) can help change relationship patterns. If your job isn't really you, try to find a way of changing to one which reflects your core values more closely. This will be far more fulfilling.

If you are thinking you are too old to make these kinds of changes, let me reassure you it is never too late to 'come home to yourself' and start leading an authentic life. I have witnessed hundreds of people who, at all ages, when confronted with the diagnosis of cancer have made key changes to their lives and in the process have literally come back to life in spirit, mind and body, restarting their lives on much better foundations.

SPIRITUAL NOURISHMENT

The next vital step is to find ways of nourishing your precious and beautiful spirit. Having read the last few pages, your spirit may already be jumping for joy at the thought of getting some recognition and attention, and being given permission to fully express yourself in life.

Many people grow up thinking spirit equals religion, and experience religion as something which represses rather than frees their spirit. Historically, the other sad thing about religious practice in the West is that spirituality has been something that is acknowledged perhaps once a week, on a Sunday, as opposed to continuously in our lives. His Royal Highness the Prince of Wales, in his millennium Reith lecture, urged people to 'rediscover or reacknowledge a sense of the sacred in our dealings with the natural world and with each other'. By doing this we live spirituality as opposed to keeping it in a separate compartment of our minds.

Buddhists and yogis believe that the material world and even our emotions are an illusion and that it is the spiritual dimension which is reality. They maintain that it is our preoccupation with the material world and our sense of self which stops us from understanding the real nature of this reality and from experiencing the associated bliss and freedom.

Recognition of the spiritual dimension of life has reached unprecedented levels in our culture at this time. People changing from material to spiritual values are often described as being 'in transformation'. The difference is very obvious when you meet people who are no longer in the grip of material values and the anxiety that goes with them. Invariably, these people say that the only thing to live for is the present moment and that when this can be given full loving attention, life becomes truly happy.

Mair Hoskins was diagnosed in 1998 with a very aggressive cancer which had already spread to her lymph nodes. She was offered radiotherapy treatment and was advised by her consultant to 'go home and live every day as if it was your last'. She was shocked and put into deep despair by his words.

Her radiotherapy involved her staying at the oncology centre in Bristol for five weeks. She had always had a gift for drawing but had not developed it. She had been on a pastel painting course earlier in the year but had been too busy to follow it up. Now with so much time on her hands, waiting for appointments, she had the perfect opportunity to paint. She filled her time with painting and carried on painting when she got home. At first it had been an experiment with the pastels, just to occupy her time so she did not have to think about the cancer. But soon it became a great joy to her. She even managed to sell two of her pictures to raise the money to go to the Bristol Cancer Help Centre for a week with her husband. A year later, in November 2000, she wrote:

> *The experience of Bristol was to change my life. As soon as I walked through the doors of the Centre I was greeted with such love and care from all the staff. There was nothing formal or intimidating about the Centre. There was a relaxed loving atmosphere that immediately put me at ease. Before, I had felt helpless about my situation but gradually I began to feel more in control. There was something I could do for myself to improve my chances of survival. Changing my diet and eating healthy, healing foods was just the beginning. I became more aware of the whole of me – of my body, mind and spirit, and getting them working together in harmony.*

Through meditation, relaxation and visualization I began to find a peace within myself.

On the Wednesday night of my week at Bristol, Pat Pilkington, one of the Centre's original founders, led us in a group healing meditation. During the meditation I had a very special experience of God's love for me, and such an infilling of His Spirit that the joy I felt was inexpressible. It was an overwhelming and life-changing experience. And the joy is still with me over a year later. I can honestly say that the happiness I felt then, I still feel now. I was brought out of a place of dark despair into the healing light of God's love. It has given me a burning desire to help and encourage others going through similar times of crisis and challenge.

Before I had cancer, I was too busy to do the things I really wanted to do. I rushed about, not stopping long enough to appreciate the beauty around me and was always looking forward to the next project. Now I am living my life moment by moment, savouring the little things that I once took for granted, experiencing all the wonderful things around me and expressing my joy in the art form that I love.

I have so much to be grateful for – all the staff at Bristol and their loving care and the strategies they gave me in my fight against cancer, the love and support of a wonderful husband, my children, all my family and friends, the prayers of a supportive Church – and, most of all, the assurance of God's love for me which I received that night at the Bristol Cancer Help Centre.

I have witnessed this transformational process over and over again at the Cancer Help Centre in Bristol, as the shock of a cancer diagnosis awakens people to the reality of their spiritual nature. For others, fleeting glances of their spiritual nature and connection to life can come at moments of intense joy, pain or beauty, through sexual union with another, whilst meditating or through experiencing true communion with God or the Holy Spirit. Sometimes people reach this state under the influence of consciousness-raising drugs. What is most important is the recognition that each of us has our own way of experiencing our own spirit and the spiritual dimension, and it is finding ways of exploring this for yourself which is the key.

As we explore our spiritual life we are presented with the paradox that on the one hand we must be individual and express our true nature, whilst on the other hand we must learn to 'let go and let God'. To be fully in the world whilst retaining our sense of the greater spiritual reality and our ability to let go into the bigger Truth, is the challenge 'to be in the world but not of it'.

The appreciation of these different levels of reality comes from a shift in our perception or consciousness. In everyday consciousness, we need our ego, a strong sense of self and the will to live out our unique purpose. But from time to time we 'get above the clouds' and see the greater reality, appreciating the tiny part we play in the vast process of life. From this perspective, the pressures and priorities of our own existence become quite unimportant. Once you have experienced this other perspective, you will not let your life be so driven or stressed, or get so lost in your 'personal drama', and will perhaps even stop taking yourself quite so seriously!

When developing individual spirituality, it is also

important to be completely authentic. People can spend years going to church or sitting in meditation groups following other people's 'recipes' for the spiritual life, feeling absolutely nothing at all. If you are doing this, I suggest you stop straightaway and do something more profitable with your time.

As I have watched people unfold into their own sense of spirit and spirituality, I have noticed recurring themes. One universal source of spiritual uplift is beauty, and the aim is to bring more and more beauty into life, whether this be through nature, the home, clothes, art or exquisite music. In Japan, there is a group called the Johrei Society whose fundamental philosophy is that health depends on three things – respect for the environment and eating organic food, daily spiritual healing within the family context, and the central place of beauty in life. Before coming across this group, I had never seen the need for beauty expressed so strongly, but the more I think about it, the more I agree that beauty in our lives is central to our spiritual health. If people live in an ugly, concrete jungle, they can become starved of the uplift that natural beauty offers. Making time to catch the dawn or climbing to the top of a mountain to see for miles around, can be deeply uplifting to our spirit.

Another key to spiritual nourishment is simply taking time and space for yourself, as has been mentioned over and over again in this book. Often, the spirit longs for simplicity and time to 'be' rather than 'do'. If you find it impossible to rest or have space in your own home, it may be worth going on retreat. There are more and more centres where it is possible to have time to yourself in a supported, loving atmosphere, either with or without spiritual guidance. Taking regular time to come home to yourself in this way and deepening your own sense of spiritual connection is profoundly healing and nurturing and is the best possible form of preventive medicine you can give yourself.

If you already have a strong sense of spirit or are of a particular religious faith, you may wish to seek a context that supports your beliefs. But there are also plenty of atheist retreat centres around for those who wish to explore their own sense of their spirituality (see Appendix 1). Many retreat centres allow people to study or deepen meditation techniques. Doing this in a dedicated way with the support of others can make it easier to maintain the practice at home.

The most fundamental spiritual value of all is the need to give and receive love – in our personal relationships and in our relationship to God or Spirit. For some, their spiritual problem is that they have a great deal of love to give but no way of expressing it, while others feel desperately in need of love and attention. If your ability to give and receive love feels blocked, or you have simply been deprived of love through social circumstances, it is a very good idea, either through therapeutic relationships, support groups, or spiritual healing, to start to find ways of giving and receiving love in a safe context.

Many self-development groups' work courses have a strongly supportive loving ethos. It is amazing how people on these courses can receive such high-quality love and support from people who were total strangers only a few days earlier. People tend to get very stuck with the idea that, to be meaningful, love must come from a partner, close friends or family. But happily, as more and more ways to develop trust and meaningful connection with others open up, this no longer has to be the case, and a much more open sense of being part of a universal family can develop. Very good feeling is generated in yoga groups, meditation classes, support groups, tantric yoga groups and a whole host of other psychological growth and developmental workshops (see Appendix 1). As with finding the right therapist, it is always wise to vet group facilitators for their skill, experience, warmth and professionality, taking note of their reputation before signing up to courses.

For many people, a very important outlet for their love and care can be voluntary work. If, for example, you feel frustrated because all your children have left home and you are without a good partner, it can be deeply satisfying to work with those in need of loving care within the community. But try to balance the love you give out with the love you give to yourself and receive from others.

A completely different way of generating and expressing love is through Buddhist meditation called *metta bharvana* (pronounced parvana), through prayer or through absent healing. *Metta bharvana* involves sitting in meditation and gradually focusing attention on the heart area. First, you generate loving feelings towards someone you find easy to love, like a child, parent or partner. Then, gradually visualize extending your love to a wider circle of family and friends. Next, you extend the loving feeling to your colleagues and associates. You then extend this feeling to the whole community or town you live in, then to your county, country and so on. If you feel able, you then extend this feeling of compassion right around the world, until you are literally holding the world in your heart. As you get more comfortable with this practice, you can consciously include people you dislike or have feuds with, holding them in your heart until you can genuinely extend love towards them. It is also an ideal opportunity to include yourself in this process as a recipient of your own love.

Developing this sense of compassion for yourself and others will make the process of forgiveness and living in harmony much easier. When you work on this inner plane, you are rapidly changing the template or programme with which you live the whole of your life. Once you start to hold your enemies in compassion, your relationship with them will very quickly change. And holding yourself in this compassionate way is the quickest way to develop a better relationship with yourself too. This will make adopting all the health-promoting changes suggested in this book far, far easier.

CHAPTER 6: GETTING STARTED

Having read this far you may well be feeling quite daunted or overwhelmed by the number of things you need to think about and do in order to reduce your risk of cancer. However, for most of us the most important areas to address are eating healthy food, giving up smoking, drinking in moderation, taking exercise and reducing stress. This may still sound like an awful lot, and it may be that ultimately you will need to address all of these areas, but try to start with the one which you think is the biggest offender in your case. First of all make a very clear intention to change, and get all the necessary support you need to succeed in making that change. As you see yourself making progress, tackle the next area and carry on step by step until you are in good health. Remember what has been emphasized all the way through the book – that if you are currently low in energy and emotionally vulnerable, you will need emotional support to make the changes, maybe through healing or energy medicines, before moving into self-help activity.

It is very important not to get paranoid about getting cancer because, as stressed in the mind–body section, our state of mind is very important to the state of our immune system and overall health. You will not help yourself by getting into a state of anxious preoccupation about the whole subject. The best way is to make the process of reducing your risk as enjoyable as possible, involving friends, colleagues or members of your family.

If you lose your way, do not be hard on yourself but, rather, pick up the book again and see what steps you can take to gently get yourself back on track.

If you do feel defeated, it may be time to seek the help of a holistic doctor to guide and support you through the process of preventing cancer. Many holistic doctors, like myself and others who have specialized in the holistic treatment of cancer, will be more than delighted to provide the necessary support, encouragement and guidance for anyone who wishes to address this area.

Once you are healthier and happier with a strong immune system and good diet, you will be at lower risk from environmental hazards. But continue to take good care of yourself – protect yourself in the sun and around chemicals, medicines and electromagnetic radiation, and practise safe sex.

When you have got your personal act together, it is then time to get active socially and environmentally. It is vital that all of us who are concerned about this subject begin to get vociferous about the adoption of anti-cancer policies in all areas of life. A good place to start is making sure our children and the generations that follow can eat balanced healthy diets, get safe nutritious food and live in a smoke- and pollution-free environment. We must then act to clean up our environment and work hard to restore the extraordinary planet on which we live to its exquisitely beautiful natural state.

We cannot wait for governments to act. We must all resolve to make thinking about and eradicating cancer one of our most urgent priorities. In tackling this issue we will also be confronting many of the other problems that wreck lives and cause immeasurable human suffering.

Please wake up now to the urgent need to take action. Commit yourself today to getting involved in cancer prevention. Grasp this nettle, first in your own life and then as part of a wider cancer-prevention movement, so that our grandchildren may look back on cancer as a nasty bit of history. Never has there been a clearer indication that we have drifted off course than the fact that the cells of our bodies are mutating and growing out of control. Never has there been a greater imperative to act to restore health and balance to ourselves and to our beautiful but endangered planet.

APPENDIX 1

HOLISTIC DOCTOR

Dr Rosy Daniel
The Harley Street Clinic
Oncology Unit
81 Harley Street
London
W1N 1DE
Cancer patient inquiries only telephone 020 7299 9428

CANCER CARE

Bristol Cancer Help Centre
Grove House
Cornwallis Grove
Clifton
Bristol
BS8 4PG
Centre Information: 0117 980 9500
Telephone Helpline: 0117 980 9505
Website: www.bristolcancerhelp.org
Registered Charity No: 284881

CANCER AND CANCER RESEARCH INFORMATION

Imperial Cancer Research Fund (ICRF)
Tel: 020 7269 3613
Institute of Cancer Research
Tel: 020 7352 8133
Cancer Research Campaign
Tel: 0800 226237

GENETIC CANCER SCREENING

ICRF family cancer clinics:

Yorkshire Regional Genetics Service
Department of Clinical Genetics
St James's University Hospital
Beckett Street
Leeds LS9 7TF
Tel: 0113 2837072

South Thames Regional Genetics Centre (East)
Division of Medical and Molecular Genetics
5th, 7th and 8th Floors, Guy's Tower
Guy's Hospital
St Thomas Street
London SE1 9RT
Tel: 020 7955 4648/4649

Cancer Genetics Clinics
Churchill Hospital
Headington
Oxford
OX3 7LJ
Tel: 01865 226048

USEFUL ORGANIZATIONS, PRODUCTS AND PRACTITIONERS

Acupuncture

British Acupuncture Council
Tel: 020 8735 0400

Alcoholism

Alcoholics Anonymous
Tel: 0117 9265520

Bio-energy measuring

Scenar device (available from Life Energies)
Tel: 01725 513129

Chi gong

Zhi Xing Wang
Tel: 020 7229 7187

Counselling

Centre for Transpersonal Psychology
Tel: 020 7935 7350
British Association of Counsellors
Tel: 01788 578328

Dowsing

The GEO Group
www.geo.org/dowse1.htm
Ann and Roy Procter
Tel: 01458 223215

Growth and personal development

The Centre for Transpersonal Psychology
Tel: 020 7935 7350
The Findhorn Foundation
Tel: 01309 691653

Healing

National Federation of Spiritual Healers
Tel: 0891 616080

Healing the emotions of the past

The Order of Love
Tel: 020 7359 3000
Hoffman Quadrinity Process
Tel: 001 415 485 5220 (in USA for British contacts)

Homeopathy

Society of Homeopaths
Tel: 01604 621400

Massage and lymph drainage

Massage Therapy Institute Register
Tel: 0117 661008

Meditation

Transcendental Meditation
Tel: 0990 143733
Friends of the Western Buddhist Order
Tel: 0117 9249991

Menopause

Progesterone HRT cream (available from Higher Nature, tel: 01435 883484)
Menopausal Herb Formula, Agnus Castus and Black Canosh (available from Argyll Herbs, tel: 01934 863353)

Mobile phone protection

RADAR electromagnetic stabilizer
Tel: 001 858 793 9230 (USA)

Nutrition

The Institute of Optimum Nutrition
Tel: 020 8877 9993
British Dietetic Association
Tel: 0121 6164900
The Nutrition Foundation
Tel: 020 7404 6504
The Nutrition Society
Tel: 020 7602 0228

Obesity

The Obesity Resource Information Centre
Tel: 01454 616 798
(a division of ASO: www.aso.org.uk)
The International Obesity Task Force: www.iotf.org
Weight Watchers
Tel: 0845 712 3000

Relationship problems

Relate
Tel: 01788 573241

Relaxation

Relaxation for Living
Tel: 01932 227826

Retreat centre

Sacred Space Foundation
Tel: 01786 898375

Shiatsu

Shiatsu Society
Tel: 01788 555051

Smoking

Quit line
Tel: 0800 002200

Tai chi

Rising Dragon Tai Chi
Tel: 01432 840282

Tantra

Leora Lightwoman
Tel: 020 7794 7866
Skydancing UK
Tel: 01736 759050

Vitamin and mineral level testing

Biolab
Tel: 020 7636 5959

Vitamins, minerals,
herbs and plant food extracts

Nature's Own Vitamins
Tel: 01684 310099
Bristol Cancer Help Centre Shop
Tel: 0117 9809504
Carctol (available from Mrs Yashu Amlani, tel: 0117 9736052)
Argyll Herbs
Tel: 01934 863353
IP6 and MGN3 food concentrates (available from The Nutri Centre tel: 020 7436 5122)

Yoga

British Wheel of Yoga
Tel: 01529 306851
Tessa Morgan yoga tape, for those limited physically (available from Bristol Cancer Help Centre, tel: 0117 9809504)

BOOKS

Cancer prevention

Reducing the Odds: A Manual for the Prevention of Cancer, Professor Gabriel Kune (Allen & Unwin)

Anti-cancer nutrition

The Breast Cancer Prevention and Recovery Diet, Suzannah Olivier (Michael Joseph)
Healing Foods, Dr Rosy Daniel (Thorsons)
The Detox Manual, Suzannah Olivier (Simon & Schuster)
Raw Foods, Leslie Kenton (Vermillion)
Say No to Cancer, Patrick Holford (Piatkus)
The Optimum Nutrition Bible, Patrick Holford (Piatkus)
Your Life in Your Hands: Understanding, Preventing and Overcoming Breast Cancer, Jane Plant (Virgin)

Healthy Cookery or Recipe Books

Eastern Vegetarian Cookery, Madhur Jaffrey (Jonathan Cape)
Healing Foods Cookbook, Jane Sen (Thorsons)
Hom's Vegetarian Cookery (Chinese), Ken Hom (BBC Books)
Italian Vegetarian Cookery, Paola Gann (Optima)
Leaves From Our Tuscan Garden, Janet Ross (Penguin)

Emotional and spiritual health

The Journey, Brandon Bays (Thorsons)
Life Lessons, Elizabeth Kubler-Ross and David Kessler
(Simon & Schuster)
Molecules of Emotion, Candace Pert (Simon & Schuster)
Something More, Sarah Ban Breathnach (Transworld)

Household carcinogens

The Safe Shopper's Bible, David Steinman and Samuel
Epstein (Macmillan)

The holistic approach to cancer

Living with Cancer, Dr Rosy Daniel (Robinsons)

APPENDIX 2

1 CHEMICALS IN THE ENVIRONMENT KNOWN TO DISRUPT THE ENDOCRINE SYSTEM:

- Cadmium
- DDT and its degradation products
- Di-(2-ethyl hexphtalate) (DEHP)
- Dicofol
- EBDC fungicides
- hexachlorobenzene (HCB)
- Kelthane
- Kepone
- Lead
- Lindane and other hexachlorocyclohexane congeners
- Mercury
- Methoxychlor
- Octachloro styrene
- PCB congeners (some)

- Synthetic pyrethroids

- Triazine herbicides

- 2, 3, 7, 8-TCDD and other dioxins

- 2, 3, 7, 8-TCDDF and other furans

- Tributyltin and other organotin compounds

- Alkyl phenols (non-biodegradable detergents and antioxidants present in modified polystyrene and PVCs)

- Styrene dimers and trimers

2 CHEMICALS CONTAINED IN HOUSEHOLD PRODUCTS WHICH ARE EITHER CARCINOGENIC (AFFECTING THE CELLS OF THE BODY) OR TERATOGENIC (AFFECTING THE 'GERM' CELLS, I.E. THE CELLS OF THE SPERM AND OVARIES):

CHEMICAL	EFFECT	FOUND IN
Acetoxyphenylmercury	Teratogenic	Paints
Acid Blue 9	Carcinogenic	Toilet bowl cleaners and deodorizers
Aluminiumsilicate	Some evidence of carcinogenicity in the dry state	Some paints
Artifical coal tar colours which contain lead and arsenic	Carcinogenic	Black and brown hair dyes
Benzene	Carcinogenic	Some adhesives
Bronopol	Breaks down to formaldehyde, which is carcinogenic	Cosmetics
Cadmium	Carcinogenic and teratogenic	Some artists' oil colours
Cobalt	Carcinogenic	Some artists' oil colours

CHEMICAL	EFFECT	FOUND IN
Crystalline silica	Carcinogenic in the dry state	Cleansers, cat litter, powdered flea-control products
1, 4-dichlorobenzene (para-dichlorobenzene)	Carcinogenic	Moth repellents, toilet deodorizers
Dichlorvos (DDVP)	Carcinogenic Teratogenic	Some no-pest strips Flea collars and pet-flea-control products
Diethanolamine (DEA)	Reacts with nitrites to form nitrosannes, which are carcinogenic	Wide range of household cleaning products, cosmetics
Dioctyl phthalate	Carcinogenic	Adhesives and correction fluid
Ethoxylated alcohols	May be contaminated with 1, 4-dioctane, which is carcinogenic	Cosmetics
Formaldehyde	Carcinogenic	Some furniture polishes, cleaners, waxes and a wide range of consumer items, especially paints and related products
Hexachlorobenzene (HCB)	Carcinogenic	Some artists' oil colours

CHEMICAL	EFFECT	FOUND IN
Hydramethylnon	Carcinogenic	Some household and garden pesticides
Lanolin (may be contaminated with DDT, dieldrin, lindane, diazinon and other pesticides)	Carcinogenic	Cosmetics and body and hand creams
Lead	Carcinogenic	Some artists' oil paints
Medium aliphatic-hydrocarbons	Some evidence suggesting carcinogenicity	Some car waxes
Methoxychlor	Limited evidence of carcinogenicity	Some pet-flea-control products
Methyl chloride (dichloromethane)	Carcinogenic	Some paint strippers and spray paints
Morpholine	Reacts with nitrites to form carcinogenic nitrosamines	Some furniture polishes
Naled	Transformation products include dichlorvos, which is carcinogenic	Some pet-flea-control products
Ortho phenylphenols	Probably carcinogenic	Some air fresheners and disinfectants

CHEMICAL	EFFECT	FOUND IN
Padimat-O	Can cause the formation of nitrosamines, which are carcinogenic	Sun screens and cosmetics
Permethrin	Carcinogenic	Some household and garden pesticides and pet-flea-control products
Petroleum distillates, hydrocarbons, process oils, solvents and spirits	May contain traces of benzene, which is carcinogenic	Some furniture polishes
Polychlorinated biphenyls (PCBs)	Carcinogenic and teratogenic	Some artists' oil paints
Propylene oxide	Carcinogenic	Some adhesives
Rotenone	Carcinogenic	Some pet-flea-control products
Sodium 2,4-dichloro-phenoxyacetate	Carcinogenic	Herbicides in lawn-care products
Sodium ortho-phenylphenol	Carcinogenic	Some bathroom cleaners

CHEMICAL	EFFECT	FOUND IN
Solvent orange 3 dye Solvent red 4 dye; Blue 1; Green 3; D and C red 33; F, D and C yellow 5; F, D and C yellow 6	Carcinogenic	Some polishes Cosmetics
Talc	Carcinogenic when inhaled	Cosmetics and some household and garden pesticides
Tetrachloroethylene (perchlorethylene)	Carcinogenic	Some spot removers
Tetrachlorvinphos	Carcinogenic	Some pet-flea-control products
Titanium dioxide	Limited evidence of carcinogenicity	Some paints and shoe polishes
Triethanolamine (TEA)	Can react with nitrites to form carcinogenic nitrosamines	Some liquid all-purpose cleaning products, metal polishes, spot removers and other household cleaning products, and cosmetics
Trisodium nitrylotriacetate	Carcinogenic	Some bathroom cleaning products

3 OCCUPATIONAL CANCER RISK FACTORS

Susceptible Workers	Likely Carcinogenic Agent	Risk
Asbestos workers, miners, shipyard workers, insulaters, rubber tyre plant workers, demolition workers, brake liners	Asbestos fibres	Mesothelioma; cancer of the lung and pharynx (throat)
Brick and ceramic manufacture/workers	Arsenic, beryllium and chromium	Cancer of the skin, lung, nose, throat and liver
Cadmium production workers, metal workers, electroplaters	Cadmium	Cancer of the lung and prostate
Chemical industry workers	Amino-biphenyl, Benzene, Benzidine, Chloromethyl ether, Cadmium, Chromium, 2-naphthylamine	Leukaemia, Cancer of the pancreas, Cancer of the bladder, Cancer of the lung, Cancer of the prostate, Cancer of the throat

Susceptible Workers	Likely Carcinogenic Agent	Risk
Chromium and alloy production workers	Chromium and chromium compounds	Cancer of the lung, nose and pharynx (throat)
Coal, gas and shale oil production workers	Aromatic hydrocarbons	Cancer of the lung, skin, bladder and pancreas
Coke plant workers	Coke-oven gases and vapours	As above
Copper production smelters, electrolysers	2-naphthylamine	Cancer of the bladder and pancreas
Dye industry workers	Aminebiphenyl, benzidine and 2-naphthylamine	Cancer of the bladder and pancreas
Electrical/electronic workers, electricians, radio/TV repairers, telephone and computer mechanics	Electromagnetic Fields (EMF), beryllium	Leukaemia; lymphomas; cancer of the brain and bladder
Electroplaters/Electrolysers	Cadmium and 2-naphthylamine	Cancer of the prostate, bladder and pancreas
Farmers and agricultural workers	Ultraviolet radiation, pesticides/ weed killers	Leukaemia; lymphoma; soft tissue sarcoma; cancer of the skin, lip, prostate and lung

Susceptible Workers	Likely Carcinogenic Agent	Risk
Garage and transport workers	Diesel exhaust	Cancer of the lung
Glass manufacture workers	Arsenic, chromium compounds	Cancer of the skin, lung, liver, nose and throat
Hairdressers	Hair dyes	Cancer of the bladder
Insulators	Asbestos fibres	Mesothelioma; cancer of the lung and pharynx (throat)
Leather and shoe industry workers	Benzene, isopropyl	Leukaemia; cancer of the sinuses
Nickel production workers	Nickel 2-naphthylamine	Cancer of the nose, bladder and pancreas
Nuclear power workers	Beryllium cadmium	Cancer of the bladder, lung and prostate
Office workers	Tobacco smoke	Cancer of the lung and throat
Painters	Painting materials, benzene	Leukaemia; cancer of the lung
Petroleum workers	Arsenic, benzene and petroleum	Leukaemia; cancer of the skin, lung, gall bladder and bile duct

Susceptible Workers	Likely Carcinogenic Agent	Risk
Plastics industry workers	Vinyl chloride	Lymphomas; cancer of the liver and lung
Radiologists/radiographers, nurses	Ionizing radiation, cancer drugs	Leukaemia; myeloma; cancer of the skin, thyroid, brain, lung, breast, bone and pancreas
Rubber tyre manufacture workers	Asbestos fibres, benzene, auramine and 2-naphthylamine	Mesothelioma; leukaemia; cancer of the lung, bladder, pancreas, gall bladder and bile duct
Steel workers	Coke-oven gases and vapours	Cancer of the lung and kidney
Tanners	Arsenic	Cancer of the skin and lung
Uranium miners	Ionizing radiation and radon gas	Leukaemia; myeloma; cancer of the skin, thyroid, brain, lung, breast, bone and pancreas
Waiters/bar tenders	Tobacco smoke	Cancer of the lung and pharynx (throat)
Woodworkers, carpenters, furniture makers, polishers and finishers	Wood dust and benzene	Leukaemia; cancer of the nose, sinuses and pharynx (throat)

4 RISK FACTORS FOR SPECIFIC CANCERS:

Anal cancer

- genetic inheritance
- the sexually-transmitted infection human papillomavirus (HPV)
- anal and genital warts caused by genital herpes (*Herpes simplex* type II).
- anal fissures and fistulas
- anal intercourse
- immunosuppressive drugs
- smoking (possibly)

Bladder cancer

- smoking
- pain killers containing phenacetin (now withdrawn from sale)
- bladder papilloma
- artificial sweeteners (possibly)
- high coffee consumption

- recurrent bladder infections

- radiation to the pelvis

- occupational exposure to aromatic amines, paints, hair-dressing products, printing products

Cancer of the bowel

- genetic inheritance (15 per cent of cases are inherited)

- a high-calorie diet with excess fat and sugar, meat (especially red) and salt

- a diet low in vegetables, fruit, fibre, fish and calcium

- being overweight

- physical inactivity

- high alcohol consumption (more than three units a day for men and two units a day for women) over a period of twenty years

- smoking (thought to account for 10 per cent of bowel cancers)

Brain tumours

- genetic inheritance (in association with neurofibro-matosis)

- use of pesticides and insecticides

- exposure to petrochemicals, rubber and vinyl chloride; electromagnetic fields (in electrical and electronic industry workers); radiation (in radiologists and radiographers) and uranium (in uranium miners)

- head injuries (slightly increased risk of meningioma)

- excessive number of dental X-rays (slightly increased risk of meningioma and glioma)

- nitrate-containing foods, e.g. sausages and salamis

- smoking (possibly)

- exposure to low-frequency electromagnetic fields from living or playing near to high-tension electricity wires (possible risk for children)

Breast cancer

- genetic inheritance

- alcohol (more than two units a day)

- high hormone levels due to obesity, diet, HRT or the Pill (and possibly environmental oestrogen mimicking substances called xeno-oestrogens)

- physical inactivity

- excessive radiation of the chest

- a high-calorie diet with excess meat and fat

- obesity

- low vegetable and fibre intake

Cervical cancer

- infection with the human papillomavirus (HPV) and genital warts virus *Herpes simplex* type II

- abnormalities in the mucous membrane of the cervix (CIN 1, 2 and 3)

- abnormalities in the mucous membrane of the vagina or skin of the vulva

- unsafe sex

- smoking

- a diet low in vegetables, fruit, betacarotene, vitamin C and folic acid

Gall bladder cancer

- genetic inheritance where there is a tendency to cholesterol gallstones (gallstones are more common with multiple pregnancies, obesity, a high-calorie diet and a diet low in fruit, vegetables and cereals)

- gallstones, especially if they are big and the gall bladder wall is calcified

- occupational exposure to products used in the car manufacturing, petroleum, rubber and textile industries

Kidney cancer

- genetic inheritance in association with non-polyposis colorectal cancer syndrome

- occupational exposure to leather, dyes, textile dyes, rubber, plastic, coke ovens, cadmium, asbestos, petroleum, tar and pitch products

- phenacitin pain killers (now withdrawn from sale)

- some diuretics and anti-hypertensive drugs and diet pills

- kidney injury

- radiation

- long-term haemodialysis

- large kidney stones

- smoking

- being overweight

Leukaemias

- genetic inheritance (very rarely, but higher risk in those with Down's syndrome)

- occupational exposure to products used in the chemical industry, shoe trade and uranium mining; exposure to the solvent benzene (also found in unleaded fuel), radiation and low-frequency electromagnetic fields (in electrical and electronic industry workers) and pesticides (in farmers)

- previous radiation exposure from diagnostic X-rays or radiotherapy

- chemotherapy with melphalan and chlorambucil

- the antibiotics chloramphenical and phenylbutazone

- smoking (possibly)

Liver cancer

- alcohol (intake of more than two to three units a day)

- smoking (possibly)

- genetic inheritance (very rarely)

- past hepatitis B and hepatitis C infection

- exposure to aflatoxin in tropical countries (especially Africa)

- chronic liver disease, e.g. liver cirrhosis

- previous steroid use, especially androgenic anabolic steroids

- oral contraceptives (possibly)

- previous blood transfusion

Lung cancer

- smoking, which causes 85 per cent of lung cancers. About one in five people now living in developed countries will be killed by tobacco unless smoking habits change. This amounts to 250 million people, or the entire population of the United States. Most alarming is the increase in female deaths from smoking. Lung cancer has overtaken breast cancer as the major cause of death among women in Scotland and northern England and may soon be the case in the whole of the UK. In Britain, smoking causes 100,000 deaths every year, 50,000 of which are due to cancer. This is the same as a jumbo jet crashing every day and killing all of the passengers on board

- chronic lung disease

- excessive radiation of the chest

- passive smoking

- asbestos

- radon gas. The average level of radon gas in the UK is 20 bequerels per cubic metre. At a level of 200 bequerels per cubic metre the risk of lung cancer is 20 per cent higher. At 400 bequerels per cubic metre the increase is around 40 per cent. Radon is believed to be responsible for 5 per cent of lung cancers in Britain

- occupational exposure to nickel and chromium compounds and arsenic

- occupational exposure to asbestos (especially in those who smoke)

- a diet low in vegetables

- a diet high in meat and fat

Lymphomas

Hodgkin's lymphoma
- genetic inheritance

- Occupational exposure to tar and benzene (in wood-workers, rubber workers and chemical workers)

- tonsil removal

- amphetamine usage

- use of the drug phenytoin in epilepsy (possibly)

- viral infection in glandular fever with Epstein Barr

- immune deficiency

Non-Hodgkin's lymphoma
- genetic inheritance

- occupational exposure to chlorophenols, phenoxy acids, asbestos, benzene, radiation, uranium, low-frequency electromagnetic fields, pesticides, herbicides and fertilizers

- viral infection with Epstein Barr viruses and viruses associated with AIDS

- poor and suppressed immunity

- immunosuppressive drugs, especially after a kidney transplant

- use of the drug phenytoin for epilepsy

- radiation treatment

Melanoma

- excessive sunlight (90 per cent of cases)

- genetic inheritance (2 per cent of cases)

- compromised immune function (with co-existing leukaemia or lymphoma or when using immunosuppressive drugs, e.g. after transplants)

- radiation

- multiple skin moles

- use of sunbeds

- chronic leg ulcers

- occupational exposure to tar, asphalt, pitch, waxes, heavy oils (including shale oil) and arsenic

- a diet low in vitamin A, betacarotene and vitamin C

- high fat intake

Mouth and throat cancer

- occupational exposure to nickel and asbestos, and mustard gas (historically)
- sunlight (especially for cancer of the lip)
- leucoplakia
- radiation
- infection with Epstein Barr virus
- use of tobacco, snuff and marijuana
- alcohol
- repeated irritation or abrasions in the mouth
- a diet low in vitamins C, E and betacarotene

Cancer of the oesophagus (gullet)

- genetic inheritance
- a 'Barrett's oesophagus', a condition in which there is reflux of the contents of the stomach into the gullet, which over time causes inflammation, scarring, narrowing or out-pouching
- alcohol
- smoking
- smoked, pickled, cured and preserved foods
- low intake of betacarotene and vitamins C and E

Cancer of the pancreas

- genetic inheritance

- occupational exposure to nickel, copper and asbestos (in chemical and dye workers), uranium (in rubber workers), and radiation (in radiologists and radiographers)

- chronic pancreatitis (inflammation of the pancreas)

- diabetes (slightly increases risk)

- smoking

- a diet high in fat and meat with low vegetable and fruit intake

- high alcohol consumption

Cancer of the penis

- the sexually-transmitted infection human papillomavirus (HPV) and the genital warts virus *herpes simplex* type II

- a narrowed foreskin coupled with poor hygiene in the uncircumcized

- unsafe anal sex, risking infection of the above viruses

- occupational exposure (in farmers) to fertilizers, pesticides and weed killers

- smoking

Prostate cancer

Possible **risk factors:**

- high testosterone levels or high testosterone/oestrogen ratios

- a high-fat diet

- genetic inheritance

- physical inactivity

- smoking (which increases the testosterone/oestrogen ratio)

- occupational exposure to pesticides (in farmers) and cadmium (in battery and alloy workers and during electroplating)

- obesity

- a diet low in betacarotene and foods containing vitamin E

- low intake of green leafy vegetables

- inadequate sunlight with resulting low levels of vitamin D

- vasectomy at a young age

- smoking

However, the causes of prostate cancer are still not well understood.

Sarcomas (cancers of the bones or connective tissues)

- genetic inheritance in association with von Recklinghausen's disease (rarely)
- occupational exposure to herbicides, wood preservatives, radiation and defoliants
- Paget's disease of the bone (where cartilage grows into the bone)
- radiation and chemotherapy treatments
- HIV infection progressing to AIDS – Karposi's sarcoma
- metallic surgical implants
- bullet and shrapnel fragments in the body's connective tissue
- smoking

Stomach cancer

- family history
- type A blood group (increases the risk by 20 per cent)
- infection with the bacterium *Helicobacter pylori*
- previous surgical removal of part of the stomach (can have an effect fifteen to forty years later)
- pernicious anaemia where there is no normal stomach-acid production

- all conditions which cause low stomach acid

- a diet low in vegetables, fruit, cereals, betacarotene and vitamins C and E

- a diet high in pickled, salted or cured foods, or foods preserved in nitrate such as salami, sausages, hot dogs, smoked meat, smoked fish or pickled food (all of which cause production of carcinogenic nitrosamines in the bowel)

- smoking

Testicular cancer

- genetic inheritance (very rarely)

- occupational exposure to defoliants (in Vietnam veterans)

- undescended testicles

- mumps orchitis (inflammation of the testicles due to mumps)

- maternal use of diethylstilboestrol (banned since 1965)

- synthetic oestrogens in food

- a sedentary lifestyle

- tight trousers

Thyroid cancer

- genetic inheritance

- occupational exposure to ionizing radiation (in radiologists, radiographers and uranium miners)

- excessive alcohol consumption

- pre-existing thyroid illness

- exposure to radiation (since 1987, more than 1000 children in the Chernobyl area have developed cancer of the thyroid due to exposure to radioactive iodine after the nuclear accident)

Cancer of the uterus (womb) and ovaries

- genetic inheritance – in association with hereditary non-polyposis colorectal cancer or breast/ovarian cancer syndrome

- previous breast, colorectal, ovarian or uterine cancer

- use of oestrogen-only HRT (increases the risk of uterine cancer more than ovarian cancer)

- polycystic ovaries

- use of fertility drugs (raises ovarian cancer risk)

- tamoxifen, the oestrogen-blocking drug used to help prevent breast cancer or its recurrence (increases risk to the endometrium or lining of the womb (uterus))

- long menstrual life with periods starting before twelve and finishing after fifty years of age

- not having children

- high blood pressure or diabetes

- a high-calorie and high-fat diet

- a diet low in vegetables, fruit and fish

- being overweight

- physical inactivity

- never having used the birth control pill

Vaginal and vulval cancer

- maternal use of diethylstilboestrol (banned since 1965)

- infection with the human papillomavirus (HPV) and genital warts virus *Herpes simplex* type II

- abnormalities in the skin or mucous membrane of the vulva or vagina

- radiation treatment

- extensive sexual activity in the very young, without adequate protection (high risk of sexually-transmitted diseases)

- smoking

5 ANTI-CANCER FOODS AND THE PHYTOCHEMICALS THEY CONTAIN

Food	Phytochemicals
Alfalfa	Saponins, sterols, flavonoids, coumarines and alkaloids, vitamins and minerals
Alliums: onions, spring onions, garlic, leeks, chives	Allium compounds – diallyl sulphide and allyl methyl trisulphide
Almonds	Protease inhibitors, phytate, genistein, lignans and benzaldehyde
Apples	Chlorogenic acid and caffeic acid
Brassicas: broccoli, cabbage, Brussels sprouts, collards, kale, bok choy, kohl rabi, arugula, horseradish, radish, swede and turnip	Dithiolthiones, isothyocyanates, glucosinolates, indole-3-carbinol and sulphurophane (in broccoli)
Sprouted broccoli and cauliflower seeds	Sulphurophane (10–100 times higher levels than in the vegetables themselves)
Burdock root (gobo) – a component of the cancer remedy Essiac	Benzaldehyde, phytosterols, glycosides, mokko lactone and arctic acid

Food	Phytochemicals
Citrus fruits	Coumarines and D-limonene, hesperatin, narangenin, glutathione and bioflavinoids
Flax oil	Omega-3 fats and antioxidants
Garlic	Selenium, germanium, antioxidants, isoflavones and allyl sulphide
Ginger	Antioxidants, gingerol and carotenes
Grapes	Antioxidants and ellagic acid (raisins also contain tannins and caffeic acid)
Licorice	Triterpenoids
Linseeds	Lignans and omega-3 essential fatty acids and alpha linolenic acid
Mushrooms (maitake, rei-shi, shiitake)	Polysaccharide immune stimulants (which boost interferon and interleukin levels), selenium, antioxidants, lignans and adaptogenic compounds
Nettles	Carotenes, chlorophyll, folic acid and selenium
Fresh nuts and seeds, particularly almonds, walnuts, black walnuts, pecans, sunflower, sesame and linseed (flax seed)	Protease inhibitors, essential fats and antioxidants

Food	Phytochemicals
Olive oil	Specific antioxidants
Orange/red/purple coloured foods such as apricots, cantaloupe melons, carrots, yellow and red peppers, beetroot, squashes, sweet potatoes, red and black berries	Betacarotene and proanthocyanadins (amongst the most powerful antioxidants known)
Parsley	Phytosterols, carotenes, folic acid, chlorophyll, vitamin C, the essential oils terpenes and pinenes, and polyacetylene
Pineapple	Bromelain; protease inhibitors; citric, folic, malic and chlorogenic acids
Potatoes	Protease inhibitors, chlorogenic acid, and vitamin C
Pulses and beans	protease inhibitors, lignans, genistein and phytosetrols
Brown rice	Rice bran saccharide
Seaweeds (kombu, kelp, nori, arame, laver bread, dulse, wakame)	Antioxidants, carotenes, selenium, iodine, alginic acid, the full range of minerals and trace elements, and vitamin B12
Soy products	The isoflavones genistein and diadzein, phytic acid, saponins, phytosterols, protease inhibitors, omega-3 fats and lecithin

Food	Phytochemicals
Teas	
black tea	The polyphenols theaflavin and thearubigin (which interfere with the initiation, promotion and growth stages of cancer)
green tea	Epicatechin (the strongest antimutagen of any plant yet examined) and epigallocatechin-3-gallate
all leaf teas	Antimutagenic tannins, antioxidants and polyphenols
Tomatoes	Antioxidants, flavonoids, lycopene, chlorogenic acid, coumarines, carotenes and carotenoids
Turmeric	Curcumin

For a full explanation of the scientifically researched properties of these phytochemicals see Suzannah Olivier's book, *The Breast Cancer Prevention and Recovery Diet*.

GLOSSARY

adducts: chemical additions to DNA which distort its
   structure

adenomatous: relating to an adenoma, an outgrowth of
   the mucous membrane lining of the bowel

aflatoxin: a metabolic product of a fungus that contaminates grains stored in hot and humid conditions

aneuploidy: loss or gain of a single chromosome

apoptosis: cell death

beta-agonists: substances which stimulate beta-adrenaline
   receptors in the body

carcinogenesis: the process by which cancer develops

carcinogens: cancer-causing agents

catechins: anti-cancer substance found in green tea

cell lineage: the generations of cells descended from a
   parent cell

DNA: deoxyribonucleic acid, the main constituent of the
   chromosomes of all organisms

endocrine system: hormonal system of the body

free radicals: chemically active compounds which can
   cause DNA damage

genome: the complement of single chromosomes contained in a nucleus, i.e. half of the twenty-three pairs of chromosomes

leukaemia: disease in which white blood cells are overproduced by bone-marrow and blood-forming organs

lymphoma: a malignant tumour of the lymph nodes

melanoma: malignant tumour of melanin-forming cells (usually in the skin)

mesothelioma: cancer of the lining of the lung

metastases: secondary cancers in tissues or organs distant from the site of origin of a cancer

mind–body techniques: techniques (such as meditation, relaxation and visualization) which affect the state of mind and subsequently the state of the body

mutagens: substances which induce genetic changes that may lead to cancer

mutations: changes in DNA, the genetic material of nearly all living organisms

myeloma: disease of the bone marrow

neurotoxicity: toxicity to nerve tissue

nitrosamines: carcinogenic compounds formed from nitrites or nitrates

oncogenes: cancer genes

pharmacogenetic polymorphisms: genetic susceptibility to environmental chemicals

phytochemicals: plant chemicals that protect against cancer

polycyclic aromatic hydrocarbons: cancer-causing chemicals found in smoke

protease inhibitors: substances which inhibit the protein-
    digesting enzymes that are thought to protect cells from
    ionizing radioactivity
proto-oncogenes: genes that normally control cell growth
    and proliferation but which can become mutated in one
    or two steps, facilitating the development of a cancer
psychoneuroimmunology (PNI): the study of how the
    mind and body are linked
sarcoma: cancer of the bones or connective tissues
teratogenic: producing cancerous change in the sperm or
    egg tissues which can then be passed to offspring
toxins: cell poisons

INDEX

industrial pollution 28, 60, 145
inertia 2
infection 47, 139
intensive farming, effects of 28
International Obesity Task
    Force 98
intrauterine device (IUD) 138

Jung, Carl Gustav 268

kelp 39
kidney cancer 41, 96
kombu 39

larynx, cancer of 37, 41, 42, 51,
    60
LeShan, Dr Lawrence 77,
    247–8, 269
leukaemia 54, 55
lifestyle 1, 9, 10–11, 28
    exercise 71–4, 186, 211–14
    sedentary 29, 71–2
Lindgren, Zoe 237–9
lip, cancer of 41
liver cancer18, 36, 41, 42, 48,
    51, 86, 155
Living with Cancer (Daniel) 6
loneliness 2
lung cancer 18, 32, 36, 37, 41,
    117–18
lymph, cancer of 26, 55

McGilvray, Lynda 187–8
McGuire, Dr Ann 245–7
ME *See* myalgic
    encephalomyelitis
meal plans 198–9
Mearess, Ainsley 241
meat and animal produce 35,
    36, 101, 109–13
Medical Research Council 28
meditation 12, 107, 122, 177,
    238, 239–43, 278–9

mesothelioma (cancer of the
    lining of the lung) 18
Metta bharvana 278–9
microwaved food 58, 116
microwaves 57–8, 143
mind 76–81
    affirmation 175, 260
    'cancer personality' 76
    meditation 12, 107, 122,
        177, 238, 239–43, 278–9
    spirit 177–81, 245 (*see also*
        Chapter 5)
    Transcendental
        Meditation (TM) 243
    visualization 78, 171, 175,
        176, 238
    see also health, holistic
        approach to; immune
        system
minerals 37, 38, 208
    lack of 28
    selenium 90, 208, 209
    zinc 208
    see also diet, food and
        nutrition
mobile phones 57, 142
mouth, cancer of 37, 41, 51
mushrooms 39
mutation:
    cells 19–21
    germline 23
    somatic 23
    point 19
    chromosomes 19
    genomic 19
myalgic encephalomyelitis
    (ME) 156
myeloid leukaemia 41

nationality 42, 85
    Africa 86
    Japan 85–6
    see also under smoking 85